Lessons from Mergers

Voices of Experience

Lessons from mergers

Voices of Experience

Nancy Linenkugel

Health Administration Press
ACHE Management Series

05 04 03 02 01   5 4 3 2 1

Library of Congress Cataloging-in-Publication Data

Linenkugel, Nancy, 1950–
    Lessons from mergers: voices of experience/Nancy
    Linenkugel.
        p. cm.
    Includes bibliographical references.
    ISBN 1-56793-141-3 (alk. paper)
        1. Hospital mergers—United States. 2. Hospitals—United
    States—Staff—Interviews. 3. Hospital patients—United States—
    Interviews. I. Title.
        RA981.A2 L56 2000
        362. 1'1'0973—dc21   00-056702
                                                                      CIP

The paper used in this publication meets the minimum requirements of American National Standards for Information Sciences—Permanence of Paper for Printed Library Materials, ANSI Z39.48–1984. ∞ ™

Health Administration Press
A division of the Foundation of the
    American College of Healthcare Executives
One North Franklin Street, Suite 1700
Chicago, IL 60606-3491
312/424-2800

CONTENTS

Acknowledgments   vii

Preface   ix

1   Adjusting the Microphone   1

2   Recognizing Why Organizations Merge   11

3   Envisioning the Future: What Organizations
     Expect to Accomplish   23

4   Understanding How the Hospitals Fit Together   39

5   Creating a Governance Structure   61

6   Understanding the Postmerger Conditions   67

7   Deciding How to Handle Employees   103

8   Creating a New Identity   113

9   Understanding What Has Been Created   117

10   Evaluating the Outcome   139

11   Replaying the Tape   161

Suggested Readings   167

Acknowledgments

Gratitude is a virtue that makes society much more pleasant. A gracious author could create an enormously long list of names of those deserving to be mentioned for their contributions to a work. While I am no exception, and after much effort, I will restrict myself to thanking just a few of the many that I could thank for assistance/inspiration with this project.

- Case Western Reserve University's Weatherhead School of Management faculty members: John Aram, Ph.D., Director of the EDM Program; Jagdip Singh, Ph.D., and Gil Preuss, Ph.D., faculty advisors; friends Paul Salipante, Ph.D., Dick Boland, Ph.D., and Sue Nartker;
- Sandi Foster, John Renner, and Marlene Light at Providence Hospital;
- All the *voices* whose words brought this book to life;
- Health Administration Press' staff, who were enthusiastic about "a practitioner writing a book"; and
- Special friend, Jackie Mayer, whose own story of overcoming challenges made this book-writing effort seem a breeze.

Sister Nancy Linenkugel, OSF, EDM, FACHE
Sandusky, Ohio

Preface

I have long studied others in business situations, placing myself in those situations and asking myself, "What would I have done differently?" It has been a useful exercise over the years, and if nothing else, it has been an opportunity to tell myself that I've often been on the right track.

The business situation of a merger adds complexities to the usual business dynamics, for in a merger there is not just one manager or one board chair in the hot seat. Now counterparts vie for dominance of vision, values, and victory. That dominance also has farther-reaching tentacles, as change is felt in two organizations instead of just one.

The opportunity to study mergers on a more intimate level occurred during fieldwork I did in the fall of 1998 for my doctoral dissertation. Because this fieldwork was both qualitative and quantitative in focus, the data were more powerful than I had imagined at the outset of the project. My findings were so powerful that they could not be contained in the 500-page academic-style writing of the dissertation; they needed to be shared in another way.

This book represents that sharing. It offers the candid interview comments of many individuals who speak firsthand about life before—and after—a merger. When I conducted the interviews, it occurred to me that many of the comments would be useful to other people. Although the research was conducted in hospital settings, the experience is applicable to mergers in general.

These voices share plenty of mistakes as they explain what they would do differently the next time, but they also show much triumph, positive thought, and pride. I feel certain that if it were possible for each interviewee to stand before you in person and share his or her stories, each one would be willing, pleased, and flattered to have you ask questions about each situation. Experience is a great teacher, and a wealth of experience shines through in the following pages. I have tried to let the experts speak from their own situations, in their own voices, in *Lessons from Mergers: Voices of Experience*.

Chapter 1

ADJUSTING THE MICROPHONE

Hospitals operate in a turbulent environment. Problems of reimbursement from the government and insurance companies abound; simply put, not enough dollars are available to fund all the care and services people need or desire. Healthcare providers must become more efficient in delivering care and services. Care and services are often delivered in nonhospital settings, such as outpatient clinics or patients' homes. Consumers are more informed about matters involving their own health—for example, many talk about their cholesterol levels just like they do their weight or age—and they are demanding to be included as partners in their own care rather than as "objects" that meekly submit to doctors' orders.

These changes require nontraditional responses from hospitals. The proliferation of hospital mergers is one response to the current environment, as hospitals scramble to ensure the survival of their operations. Reasons for hospital mergers include the following:

1. Because of the overall economics of the healthcare industry, it is more difficult to be a stand-alone facility when competition for patients increases.

2. Integrated health delivery systems are often preferred by local residents, who find it easier to obtain a spectrum of healthcare services from allied, connected providers.
3. Community pressures require more value in hospital services, for example, elimination of duplication and lower costs.

The reasons that compel any business to seek merger partners apply in the hospital world, because the hospital is not only a place of care but also a place of business. A significant number of hospital mergers occurred between 1994 and 1999; the highest number occurred in 1996, when 235 deals were made involving 768 facilities.[1] In 1995, 230 deals were made, followed by 217 in 1997, 198 in 1998, 184 in 1994, and 142 in 1999. All totaled, the merger deals between 1994 and 1999 involved 3,997 facilities, which is over half the number of U.S. hospitals.

The merger/acquisition activity involving hospitals has been considerable, yet the desired economies of scale may not be materializing. *Trustee*[2] reported that

> of the hospitals that were acquired in the last two years, only seven percent have reduced or eliminated services after becoming part of a larger system.... Executives have had limited success combining clinical services following a merger. Only nine percent combined ambulatory care services, only eight percent combined emergency services, and eight percent combined inpatient units.

The upside of mergers is the achievement of goals for efficiency and improved services. When mergers work, they can work beautifully and be a tremendous accomplishment for the benefit of the

---

1 Bellandi, D. 2000. "Spinoffs, Big Deals Dominate in '99." *Modern Healthcare* 30 (2): 36–44.
2 "Merger Results a Letdown to Execs." 1996. *Trustee* Sept. 3, 3.

local community. But the downside or mergers can be disruption, disillusionment, and disappointment. A former hospital CEO sheds light on the darker side:

> When our hospital was acquired by a larger one 30 miles away, we thought it was a good move. I respected the other CEO and thought he respected me, since I was staying on. I thought the guy was Theory Y, but once we completed the deal, he was really Theory X. I started to see the way he and his organization really operated. My medical staff revised its bylaws, but a couple of the revisions were overturned by the parent board. My doctors were furious! They boycotted our hospital and took their patients down the street. That's when I decided to leave. I parted amicably and negotiated a decent severance package, but my hopes had really been high to stay there, and it disgusted me to see how they really operated.

During 1995, as reported in *Modern Healthcare*,[3] sixteen "busted hospital engagements" of healthcare mergers were called off. Reasons given ranged from "city officials objected" to "philosophical differences" to "governance disputes" to "details not disclosed." The shortest duration from engagement to breakup was 1 month, the longest was 13 months, and the average was 5.1 months.

Because some hospital mergers work and others do not, executives who find themselves faced with the possibility of a merger are interested in understanding the dynamics of these situations. Although every merger is a product of variables particular to its own venue and players, some generalizations can serve as guideposts for those who have no experience with a merger—or for others who wish to arm themselves with something more than their personal experience.

---

3 Lutz, S. 1996. "Failed Mergers Offer Valuable Lessons." *Modern Healthcare* 26 (1): 54–55.

FOUNDATION

The merger phenomenon for hospitals was picking up steam in the mid-1990s at the same time I was immersed in doctoral studies. Having watched and read about hospitals going through these changes, including facilities within my own system, I was interested in learning about the differences between mergers that continue on and that seem to be successful and mergers that are not successful.

That interest led to my doctoral dissertation, "Achieving Potential in Hospital Mergers," which was completed in early 1999. Because my doctoral program was designed for "practitioner-scholars," the dissertation was an extensive applied research project as a contribution to the management literature. The project was based on data obtained using the triangulation techniques of gathering qualitative data through on-site interviews with multiple informants; gathering quantitative data and making a profile analysis of the survey instrument; and performing follow-up telephone interviews, as well as compiling a meta-ethnography from the literature.

The information gleaned from this project's interviews seemed too valuable to keep tucked away in a dissertation that looks overwhelming. I wanted to let the voices of the interviewees be heard in another way, and this book serves that purpose.

The reader needs some background to set the stage. During the fall of 1998, I conducted field research at four hospital merger sites that represented similar-sized, nonacademic, nonprofit, nongovernmental, general medical-surgical community hospitals that merged between 1994 and 1997 in which movements of people or services occurred. I selected the sites based on pretest information, including the existence of accessible satisfaction data regarding patients and employees. Although four sites might appear to have limited generalizability, the multiple informants at each site provided a deeper understanding of the issues.

My research premise was that mergers achieve their potential when two independent variables "fit"; these variables are business factors (financial conditions) and culture factors (practices and people). Community response, patient satisfaction, employee satisfaction, medical staff support, and financial performance—the dependent variables—would measure merger success. I defined a *merger* as the creation of a single entity from two in which there was movement of services or staff.

The final four field sites selected represented each of the following categories of mergers, as designated by the merger CEOS:

Better for the Business/ Better for the Employees	Worse for the Business/ Better for the Employees
Better for the Business/ Worse for the Employees	Worse for the Business/ Worse for the Employees

Merger Stabilization Model

At each of the merger sites I interviewed up to 30 persons, including board members, executives, physicians, employees, patients, and community representatives. The research model I devised, called the "merger stabilization model," is shown in Figure 1.1. My very strong feeling going into the research was that in merger decisions, significant emphasis is placed on the business factors, such as operating margins, balance sheets, and cost reductions in the community from the elimination of duplication between hospitals. I also felt that merger decisions do not put enough emphasis on making sure that the "people" aspects fit, that is, the aspects such as culture considerations, philosophies, values, and practices. In essence, I hypothesized that ignoring people spells disaster in a merger.

FIGURE 1.1 Merger Stabilization Model (Theory)

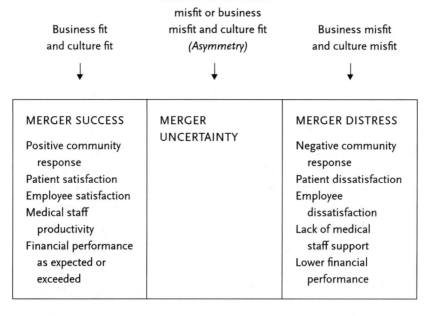

CULTURE FIT (people and community concepts)		BUSINESS FIT
Practices (intrinsic)	*Culture (intrinsic)*	Ownership
Process/results	Clan (family)	Financial performance
Employee/job	Hierarchy (structure)	Bond rating
Loose/informal	Adhocracy* (innovative)	Physical plant
Parochial/professional	Market (business)	Technology arsenal
Open/closed		Scope of services
Normative/pragmatic		Market share
Internal/market		Managed care relationships
		Days A/R
Expectations of patients and community citizens (extrinsic)		Regulatory compliance
		Tax status

Business fit and culture fit	Business fit and culture misfit or business misfit and culture fit *(Asymmetry)*	Business misfit and culture misfit
↓	↓	↓

MERGER SUCCESS	MERGER UNCERTAINTY	MERGER DISTRESS
Positive community response		Negative community response
Patient satisfaction		Patient dissatisfaction
Employee satisfaction		Employee dissatisfaction
Medical staff productivity		Lack of medical staff support
Financial performance as expected or exceeded		Lower financial performance

*Adhocracy, a term coined by Deshparde, Farley, and Webster (1993), refers to the feeling that people in an organization are loyal to their craft and thus the culture is one of putting ideas first.

In each of the mergers studied, business fit and culture fit were not enough to guarantee that the merger could achieve its full potential. The research uncovered five "process" factors emerging from the data that can affect merger potential either positively or negatively, depending on the circumstances:

1. *Time.* Time can enhance the merger through the building of trust, unfolding of the process, and growth of acceptance. Lack of time can harm the merger because of crisis motivation, hasty decision making, and too much change too fast.

2. *Transparency.* Transparency is a deliberate leadership policy that determines the public visibility of changes and consolidations. High transparency—few visible changes in the merging hospitals—is perceived by the public as the continuation of the status quo; in essence, the community keeps "its hospital." Low transparency—very apparent service consolidations and changes—can mean that service changes are perceived as "take-aways."

3. *Motivation.* Motivation is a function of the leadership's ability to transform the reasons for merging into goals and strategies for the new corporation. Motivation can enhance the merger; compellingly strong reasons for merging can carry the new fledgling organization over the initial stages despite obstacles. In contrast, when the message of why the merger is occurring gets lost, the merger can be harmed.

4. *Leadership.* Leadership can enhance the merger. The board, CEO, administration, and medical staff leaders can unite philosophically and move the merger forward—or they can harm the merger through lack of unity or inability to support decisions or see them through. Creating a new culture is a function of leadership and can carry the merger to new heights of consolidation, provided that the organization is ready and that time and attention are not consumed by operational matters that distract from this task.

5. *Proximity.* Proximity can enhance the merger or harm it. Hospitals' locations can be key determinants in service consolidation

decisions, but geographic closeness does not automatically ensure community acceptance. Merging hospitals in close proximity may be more likely to attempt service consolidations then hospitals that are located farther apart.

These factors transcend culture and business issues and focus on the circumstantial aspects of a merger. Those in the field would say, "If you've seen one merger, you've seen one merger." In other words, merger transactions are idiosyncratic.

Revised Merger Stabilization Model

Because the research showed that the factors of business fit and culture fit alone cannot guarantee that hospital mergers will achieve full potential, the model was revised to include the five process factors (see Figure 1.2.). The research data showed that the factors depicted in the model could act as on/off switches for achieving merger potential, depending on whether they have an effect before or after the merger. The two critical factors in hospital mergers achieving full potential work as follows:

1. Business fit can optimize merger potential both before and after the merger. In successful mergers, the financial strength increased; in the less-than-successful mergers, the financial distress worsened.
2. Leadership can enable mergers to reach their potential both before and after the merger. Some mergers overcome culture incompatibilities, achieve support, and create synergy. Others, in contrast, disable their potential through lack of financial planning, indecision, and inability to achieve support.

The other factors contributing to the achievement of merger potential work as follows:

FIGURE 1.2 Revised Merger Stabilization Model (Research Findings)

CRITICAL FACTORS		CONTRIBUTING FACTORS
Business Fit	Leadership • Motivation • Transparency	Culture fit Time Proximity

Factors enable achievement of full potential

Factors disable achievement of full potential

↓   ↓

MERGER SUCCESS	MERGER DISTRESS
Positive community response	Negative community response
Patient satisfaction	Patient dissatisfaction
Employee satisfaction	Employee dissatisfaction
Medical staff productivity	Lack of medical staff support
Financial performance as expected or exceeded	Lower financial performance

1. Culture fit, although enhancing the chance of merger success both before and after the merger, by itself is not powerful enough to overcome a postmerger business misfit.
2. Time enhances success when there is no premerger crisis and negatively affects success when there is postmerger crisis decision making.
3. Proximity enhances success according to community acceptance both before and after the merger. Proximity can negatively affect success depending on other postmerger aspects, such as the distance employees now must travel between the hospitals.

The revised merger stabilization model (see Figure 1.2) indicates that hospital mergers can achieve their full potential based on the critical factors of business fit and leadership, and culture fit, time, and proximity contribute to the achievement of full potential. A key finding of this research was the power of leadership as a critical factor in achieving full potential in hospital mergers. Decision makers contemplating hospital mergers need to act as one, think critically, be resolute about the decisions made, and then stick to those decisions despite the criticism or praise that ensues.

Chapter 2

RECOGNIZING WHY ORGANIZATIONS MERGE

AVOID TAKEOVER AND SURVIVE

No community wants to lose the local hospital it has relied on over the years. Hospital trustees, employees, doctors, and their patients all represent the local community through involvement with, and patronage of, their hospital. Several voices demonstrate the passion of this involvement as they defend the merger strategy as a way to avoid being taken over by other institutions:

> IT'S ANYBODY'S GUESS how long we would have survived. Our hospital was doomed to be taken over by a larger organization. We had been approached by some of the larger hospitals. But the hospital we merged with was about two and a half times smaller than we were. Probably it was doomed to be scooped up before we would have been. [board chair, successful merger]

> AS THE THREAT of mergers from outside our community came to our doorstep, we had enough people who were enlightened—who could see the handwriting on the wall. I believe their insight gave us the opportunity to say that there was a possibility we could work together. At least it was a start for a talking point.
> [trustee, successful merger]

THE BIGGEST REASON for merging, probably, is all the pressure from the outside—the bigger hospitals. The attitude was that if we didn't join and form a strong and viable alliance in the county, the bigger hospitals would acquire the rural hospitals into their own complexes. We wanted to be united so we could resist that.

[physician, successful merger]

I THINK THE merger was principally intended as a defensive measure when both hospitals saw the rapid growth of the tertiary facility. At the time the tertiary facility was very aggressive, and individually the hospitals were far more vulnerable than they would be combined.   [nursing home administrator, successful merger]

Even an employee at one of the merging hospitals, while very concerned about her own future, worried about her organization and found herself agreeing:

WE HAD TO do something. We were too small. And I definitely didn't want somebody bigger coming here and sweeping us off our feet and running us. Better to keep it right here.

[employee, successful merger]

Similar takeover-avoidance motivation was expressed by persons involved in a merger that did not pan out, although not because of any lack of passion or concerted effort:

IT SEEMED NATURAL to put the hospitals together. We were being pressed by two tertiary facilities to join them. And by *join* they meant "sell out and be acquired."   [board chair, eventual failed merger]

BOTH HOSPITALS NEEDED to be stable in the medical world. I think they did not want to be gobbled up by the tertiary facility, so they said, "Let's merge, and we'll have this corner of the county."

[employee, eventual failed merger]

In addition to the defensive posture of avoiding takeover, mergers are motivated by the need for hospitals to survive. Insolvency is not an option for community-minded decision makers who struggle to maintain open doors at their local facilities. Several patients and a community representative express a real understanding of the business situations their hospitals faced:

THE MERGER HAPPENED because one of the hospitals wouldn't have survived. The smaller one would probably be gone by now. Bigger is not always better, but smaller isn't that great, either. The hospitals all came together because they had to.

[patient, successful merger]

I WOULD IMAGINE the merger was good business sense as far as consolidating the different services that were duplicated, and they had to streamline to get operating costs down. I would imagine that one of the major reasons for the merger was to be more attractive in the financial end.

[patient, financially struggling merger]

THE REASON FOR the merger is the same as for everything else— money. I think both hospitals are in trouble. I don't understand how they could be with what they charge and everything, but I think they're both in trouble.   [patient, eventual failed merger]

THE LAYPERSON DOESN'T understand the ramifications of healthcare reimbursement, and when it's a sinking ship, how can you keep it afloat? Some things have to happen. It ain't the way it used to be.   [community representative, successful merger]

Financial survival would seem to be a very compelling reason to merge, but it was not enough to ensure the long-term success of some mergers. I vividly remember the passion of this board chairman who was the lone voice in catalyzing a merger:

THINGS WERE CHANGING more rapidly now. Managed care was starting to become a bigger threat, and everybody saw that it was going to be more difficult to stay in this business if you were alone.
[board chair, eventual failed merger]

Other comments underscore the survival motivation:

I THINK THE leaders believe they want to protect the services that we give locally. I think they felt that both hospitals could go under if they did not do something.   [employee, eventual failed merger]

I THINK BOTH our organizations were in dire straits—in a position to need to partner with somebody else.
[executive, financially struggling merger]

THE ONLY REASON the hospitals began meeting together was because they thought they'd reached the time when they couldn't survive independently.   [physician, eventual failed merger]

These voices span the spectrum of individuals in both the hospital and the community. It is not just trustees, hospital executives, or even physicians who are worried. All see a merger as one means to keep the hospital going and open.

RETAIN AUTONOMY

The entrepreneurial spirit in business is fueled by the concept of striking out on one's own, being in control, influencing one's future, and steering one's own course. One dominant theme in hospital mergers is the ability to retain an autonomous presence in a community despite competition from without. Who understands the fabric of the community's own healthcare needs better than the local providers?

Merger is sometimes seen as necessary to maintain local control and current standards:

THE OTHER HOSPITAL saw, as we did, that it was going to be hard going it alone; but they, like us, wanted to do their best to preserve local control, local governance, and these community resources.

[CEO, successful merger]

I HEARD IT at the board level: "We really have to fight to maintain control, to ensure that *we* dictate the level of healthcare in this community and that we don't allow some outside organization to come in and effectively turn our hospitals into BandAid stations and literally force our patients to go to facilities outside our community." [executive, successful merger]

THE WAY HEALTHCARE is going now, you have to rely on your neighbor a little bit to strengthen the community and your customer demographics. The tertiary facility is moving in, so if you get all your local guys working together, you can have a nice little network running and keep the big boys from the big city at bay.

[community representative, successful merger]

KEEP THE TWO hospitals as a community hospital system, and don't let them get involved in the big-city hospitals. Keep these hospitals for the people in our community, and make it a good healthcare system for them. [employee, successful merger]

Maintaining autonomy is the only way for organizations to ensure local control and the ability to decide how best to respond to local needs. Each of the following individuals might have preferred a path other than merger to achieve that autonomy, but in the end, merger provided the best hope for continued autonomy.

WE FEARED THE larger city hospital trying to pull us in. We'd rather control our own destiny. [board chair, eventual failed merger]

WE BEGAN TO sense that our board and their board were saying the same things. That realization opened the floodgates. We were not looking to control Hospital X or Hospital Y. We just wanted to keep the bad guys out. We wanted to maintain and manage our local autonomy as much as we could.

[executive, successful merger]

WE MERGED OUT of mutual need. I think the catalyst was our two CEOS talking with each other at a time when they were both aware that the marketplace was changing dramatically and systems were forming. Many people were beginning to understand that you had to be part of a broader referral system, or you were going to be left out.

[long-term care administrator, financially struggling merger]

EVEN OUR HOSPITAL isn't big enough to stay alone. But by having the partners that we do, I think we're in a better situation—a stronger situation—and we're able to keep services in our county.

[executive, successful merger]

"Going it alone" may have been the watchword for hospitals decades ago. In some locations, it still is. In others, however, the competitive business climate complicates the straightforward mission of simply providing care. Partners are needed. Various kinds of relationships form. The preservation of autonomy motivates mergers that succeed—and also those that fail.

CREATE EFFICIENCIES AND PROVIDE BETTER CARE

Creating one entity from two can have a powerful by-product: synergy. This combined energy often eclipses what the two entities could have ever hoped to accomplish single-handedly. When it is hospitals that are achieving synergy, the ability to harness purchasing power, operational efficiencies, and higher-volume patient services is a powerful impetus for merger.

Several patients interviewed had no knowledge about, or interest in, hospital mergers in their communities. A few patients, however, did offer insightful views:

I COULD SEE that if you needed a very specialized procedure that took expensive equipment, it would make sense not to have two of them but to have only one. In that sense, grouping together allows hospitals to offer more advanced technology.

[patient, successful merger]

I THINK MAYBE the hospitals would merge to be more successful in taking care of people. They'd have more power between the two than in just one hospital. They could do more with patients. There would just be more people—more power.

[patient, successful merger]

WELL, EVERYBODY THOUGHT the merger was just for money, but I don't think it was. The hospitals pooled their resources. Hospital X now has a much better cardiac care unit than Hospital Y. Hospital Y has the new neonatal unit and the cancer research center. If neither hospital has a particular facility, they can combine resources. And the smaller hospitals have someplace to refer to without a whole lot of hassle. The doctors seem to work together.

[patient, successful merger]

MAYBE, FOR EXAMPLE, the merged hospitals could have a pediatrics unit at just one hospital instead of both and save some money.

[patient, eventual failed merger]

I WOULD IMAGINE that combining the overhead expenses of the hospitals makes sense. The hospitals can group together to get better pricing for purchasing services and enlist more doctors.

[patient, successful merger]

One employee was in the unique position of holding part-time medical records jobs in each of the merging hospitals. She struggled with the contentiousness of the two facilities but decided the merger probably increased efficiency enough to allow both hospitals to coexist:

> I HOPE THEY merged because they wanted to do the best thing for the city and not lose both hospitals. I'd like to believe that's what the merger was for. I believe it was done to avoid shutting down one hospital completely.
>
> [employee, eventual failed merger]

Other employees had a similar philosophical stance:

> THEY MERGED TO provide better care for the community, and also to keep the services *in* the community. That's been said right up front. And it's one of the things that's kept us going and believing in the merger.   [employee, successful merger]

> THE MERGER, I would think, was to decrease the cost of doing business by consolidating services. And it was also to standardize our operations from a quality perspective—to adopt the better practice from each sister hospital and to benchmark to the outside.
>
> [employee, successful merger]

One physician was enthusiastic about the merger's value:

> A MUCH BETTER job could probably be done by consolidating where appropriate and saving money in those areas, trimming down those expenses, and streamlining the operation, to save money to put back into improving the healthcare to the community.
>
> [physician, eventual failed merger]

In contrast, another physician was very disappointed with the idea of merging, although admitting that there were benefits:

THERE ARE THINGS we can share very efficiently by being an affiliate. For example, both emergency rooms are supplied by the same emergency room corporation.   [physician, successful merger]

Finally, synergy was expressed in two more comments:

THE ALLIANCE BETWEEN these two hospitals was easily formed mainly because of each one's commitment to the larger community. We could really support each other in our expertise around that. Some of the other things that made it easy for these two hospitals to join were the commitment to quality service and a real commitment to holistic care.
    [community representative, financially struggling merger]

ALL WE WERE doing was looking at the other hospital and saying, "We have 60 percent occupancy, it has less; putting us together, we could manage with the number of beds we now have, and it would be very efficient."   [executive, financially struggling merger]

Synergy is a possible prize at the end of the merger trail. Whether or not it can be achieved is a function of the merger model, how the myriad merger details are handled, and the personalities involved. Behind every successful merger is a compelling reason that enables competing organizations to put aside personal agendas and create something larger and for the greater good. If that compelling reason is to create efficiencies and provide better care, the community served is the real beneficiary.

STOP COMPETING

Competing organizations may find that a compelling reason to merge is to stop the competition. As hospitals analyze the market in terms of past history and future prospects of threats, fears, and destructive duplication between competitors, they may choose collaboration over competition.

Doctors have much at stake in the decisions a hospital makes about its future. Although the merger outcomes differed, the following physicians welcomed mergers as a means to stop needless competition:

THE TWO CEOS were discussing how the market was being severely eroded by the bigger hospitals buying nearby practices: "If *we* merge and consolidate, it will make the system stronger, we can run more efficiently, and we won't overlap in the patients we have. Otherwise, we'll spend a lot of money trying to defeat one another for this common ground. Why don't we merge and protect ourselves against these folks?"   [physician, successful merger]

PEOPLE LIKE ME who have worked at both hospitals, have asked, "Why are you hospitals separate? You have common market areas, and you bite on each other. You should be working together." I guess nobody was listening until some consultants came in and said there was potential here. Both hospitals catered to the west side of town. They were targeting the same people, and forming their own practice groups—hiring doctors or buying practices. The hospitals were essentially crisscrossing their area.

[physician, financially struggling merger]

THE TWO HOSPITALS were vying for the same people. The boards finally listened to some of the physician leaders and said, "You know what? It looks like we're going to have some difficulty competing with each other. Let's talk about collaborating in some way, shape, or form."   [physician, eventual failed merger]

Board leadership can be the key to mergers that are formed to end competition:

THE COUNTY WOULD be better served by having one strong system rather than two smaller, weaker ones.

[board chair, eventual failed merger]

I TALKED TO the chair of the board of the other hospital and said, "I don't understand why we can't work out some things and at least work more closely together. If we don't, some disaster will take place, and we'll both go down the tube."

[board chair, successful merger]

Another executive understood the advantages of reduced competition in mergers because of her experience in another community:

I'M FROM A larger city. The competition there was just fierce. I did go through a merger there, and I now realize that competition is not particularly healthy within the same town.

[executive, successful merger]

Capitalist voices strike the chord that competition is the "American way" and that having choice in the marketplace is fundamentally good. Examples are numerous in daily life, with the myriad restaurants, grocery stores, automobile and clothing brands, recreational opportunities, and housing. Other voices, however, assert that capitalism is not appropriate in healthcare. Hospitals that perceive their competitive situation as unhealthy can find a solution in a merger.

Before any merger occurs, the organizations involved must agree on the reasons for the merger. In both successful and less-than-successful mergers, the parties involved clearly define why the merger is occurring. Thus, lack of purpose may not be the differentiating factor between success and lack of success in a merger. The less-than-successful merger leaders feel just as passionate about the reasons that compelled them to seek a merger partner.

It is extremely important to identify the basis for merging in the first place. However, unless the players agree on the reasons to merge, there can be no hope for a merger to achieve lift-off, let alone potentiation.

What We Have Heard

Goal	Successful Merger	Less-Than-Successful Merger
Avoid takeover and survive	yes	yes
Retain autonomy	yes	yes
Create efficiencies and provide better care	yes	yes
Stop competing	yes	yes

Clues and Hallmarks

Did you detect anything in the comments of people involved in successful mergers that indicates a greater sense of purpose or desire compared with the comments of individuals in less-than-successful mergers?

Chapter 3

ENVISIONING THE FUTURE: WHAT ORGANIZATIONS EXPECT TO ACCOMPLISH

IMPROVE QUALITY AND EXPAND SERVICES

Synergy enables entities that join to create something larger than just the sum of what each one brings to the union. A merger carries the potential for improved quality and expanded services. Achieving these potentials and any others necessitates focusing on the most positive outcomes of the partnering, rather than merely on the least negative alternatives. That sentiment was echoed by several board members whose organizations had weathered successful mergers.

> I THINK THE MAIN goal is to maintain a community health network focused on delivering care to patients here without having to send them to a major tertiary hospital. The costs are much lower in our system than other systems, so we're able to compete for the insurance end. But our goal is to provide healthcare to our community in a quality manner.   [trustee, successful merger]

> OUR GOAL WAS to improve the quality of care, bring more specialists into the community, and have people available to do things in this community so that people would not have to travel.
> [board chair, successful merger]

THE OBVIOUS PRODUCT of the whole merger experience is better quality of service to our community. Likewise, we wanted to have better-qualified physicians to carry that out.

[board chair, successful merger]

OUR INTENT WAS to work together for the betterment of the community—the community being the entire county.

[board chair, successful merger]

Executives were no less enthusiastic about a vision of improved quality and services—whether or not their mergers were ultimately poised and able to achieve it:

OUR GOAL IS to create an organization to serve the western part of our county in a far more cost-effective, efficient, and technologically improved way.   [executive, financially struggling merger]

NEW FACILITIES, NEW equipment, and therefore new supportive technologies will come from the ability to better serve our catchment area, because our facility will be state-of-the-art. We will be ten years ahead of our time. And although we'll still be a fairly small health system, we will be the future. As a result of having a far better financial foundation for growth, we can be more volume sensitive and able to incorporate economies of scale. We can thus become stronger.   [executive, financially struggling merger]

WE WILL BE serving more of the other communities in the county. We're considering doctors' offices in various other communities and looking for new business development, new areas we might be able to get into.   [executive, successful merger]

Trustees were similarly optimistic when asked about the desired outcome of their mergers. This optimism, however, was not strong enough to keep two competitors together:

OUR GOAL WAS that the residents of the metropolitan area would have quality of healthcare that was as high as they could get anyplace in the country.   [trustee, eventual failed merger]

WE WANT TO develop one strong foundation—a community foundation. That will happen. It's one of our major goals.
                              [trustee, eventual failed merger]

One employee, a nurse, had come to accept the merger itself only after she had received and analyzed information about it. Trust was an essential element for her, and she gave the administration high marks not only for offering expanded services but also for being honest and straightforward:

WE COULD OFFER patients at Hospital X the services they needed, and we could send our patients there for services we didn't provide, such as cardiac procedures. Instead of a patient going to an outside hospital, financially it's more sound for us to send the patient to another institution where we are also going to benefit financially. It's like having a sister in Florida—you can go down there and visit.   [employee, successful merger]

One of the most pragmatic interviewees was an informed person in one of the merger communities. Her opinion stood out, because so many other people in the community were either disinterested or uninformed about the fact that a hospital merger was occurring.

THE AVERAGE JOE doesn't care whether the hospitals are linked or not linked. Most people want the services to be available—to be very high quality. They want to be able to trust the hospital. The average person on the street just wants to be able to get healthcare locally and have it be great.
                       [community representative, successful merger]

One CEO's frustration was evident as he recalled the difficulty in bringing the two hospitals together. The financial aspects of that merger have not been successful to this day.

> THESE WERE TWO hospitals, and to turn one hospital into a behavioral health center or a nursing home would be quite a change. I don't think the community even knows what they have here. How do we deal with the elderly population? How do we meet their needs? How do we get them to have a relationship with our institution?   [CEO, financially struggling merger]

The lofty goal of improving care and thus expanding the services offered was shared by voices from successful and less successful mergers. It is hoped that this objective is the foundation of any hospital merger, but this goal alone cannot ensure success.

PROVIDE FOR THE COMMUNITY AND MAINTAIN AUTONOMY

No community wants to think of itself without its hospital. Decisions by hospital boards to close a facility or to be sold to an outside entity come only after agonizing deliberations and are moves bordering on desperation. One of the alternate decisions hospital boards make to retain local control is the decision for merger—a coming together of those who know the community best.

Informed physicians are invaluable in the merger process, as well as in the postmerger organizations that emerge. Two physicians describe the benefits of community-based care:

> THE MERGER IS occurring to make sure that the healthcare delivered to our service area is community based, that the resources of the community stay in the community, that the healthcare system responds to community needs, and that we still can get healthcare locally. We want to ensure that healthcare is not going to be dictated by people downtown who have a personal agenda and are

managing the healthcare of others for their own purposes. Truly and simply, the merger is to keep healthcare local.

[physician, successful merger]

OUR MERGER WAS fueled not just by mergers or acquisitions of the hospitals from the outside. There was also competition for patients from the outside, and we were striving to help keep more of the county's people in the county.

[physician, successful merger]

Executives can easily espouse local autonomy. A merger's continued financial struggle, however, poses many challenges to the executive team's faith in the decision:

WE WANT TO retain the control here. We want to have a local board that oversees the whole endeavor and not be controlled from the outside.   [executive, successful merger]

OUR OBJECTIVE IS still that of becoming what we set out to be: we want to be community hospitals in our two communities, and we want to provide the needed services. The same thing is true of our suburban campus. That's a community hospital, and we want to provide the services that people need in that setting.

[executive, financially struggling merger]

IN OUR MERGER we strive to put in place an appropriate, cost-effective delivery system for the market and to make sure that the market is served.   [executive, financially struggling merger]

THERE ARE A great number of patients in this county we're not treating yet; they're going somewhere else. Our job is to attract them here.   [executive, successful merger]

The way one community representative accepted ownership of the merger says volumes about why this merger is flourishing:

I THINK THE goals are to provide as much healthcare locally as possible and to make sure that that locally provided healthcare is clinically the very best. We also want to help those who have to go outside the community for specialized care to be prudent buyers and to still have a lot of local control over their healthcare.

[community representative, successful merger]

Two quotations from board members follow. If not noted, would you have been able to tell which merger did not stay together?

THE BASIS OF the merger was that it would benefit the people of the community to have this affiliation agreement between the two hospitals. Another, very fundamental reason for the affiliation was that it would help retain local decision making in regard to health-care delivery.   [board chair, eventual failed merger]

WE FEEL THAT if we can keep this alliance in the community, by the community, and for the community, the community is going to gain so much more, because we're doing it for ourselves. We're taking ownership of it. It's ours. It keeps us from becoming another number in some large organization's list, and it keeps us from being at their mercy.   [trustee, successful merger]

Finally, two employees agree that the mergers at their hospitals were undertaken to maintain community-based healthcare. The cynical undertone of the first statement betrays the tension and difficulties felt throughout the entire organization:

I HOPE THE merger was done to save healthcare in the area. It would be my hope, too, that it was an attempt to promote the best that we can give. I hope that's the true reason.

[employee, eventual failed merger]

THE HOSPITAL MERGED for the purpose of the customers—to keep our customers here in our community so they don't have to drive 50, 70, or 80 miles. I see a lot more people staying instead of leaving the area—my friends, neighbors, and relatives.

[employee, successful merger]

Once again, similar motivation—to maintain local autonomy in hospitals—exists in both mergers that succeed and those that have less success. Success is a result of intimate knowledge of, and insight into, internal and external market information. Creating a responsive healthcare organization within a merger vehicle can preserve an autonomous care legacy for years to come.

ELIMINATE COMPETITION AND WORK TOGETHER

If the universal mission of every hospital is quality healthcare for all, the ideal of working together would not seem excessively difficult to achieve. In reality, though, each hospital has gone about achieving its mission in its own way, with a particular philosophy, culture, and heritage. These particularities often form the basis for decades of competitive differentiation and niche segmentation between hospitals in a community, which in turn creates inadvertent, almost insurmountable barriers to collaboration. Overcoming these obstacles is another goal in mergers.

Naturally, executives feel the sting of constant competition as much as, if not more than, anyone else:

THE EXPECTATION OF the merger is to eliminate competition and to work cooperatively for the benefit of the total community.

[executive, successful merger]

THE TWO CEOS very quickly realized that it probably made more sense, as community-based organizations, to collaborate instead of compete, especially because the true competitors, or the true competitive forces, were coming out of the city. Those tertiary facilities were really moving on into the community to try and secure their patient base. When you look at where Hospital X is and where

Hospital Y is, and how we came together in our geographic area, it's kind of neat.   [executive, successful merger]

Board chairs feel the sting of competition when local residents voice their concerns about duplication of services and lack of cooperation between the hospitals. The following board chairs each attempted to fulfill their governance roles by focusing on community need rather than institutional need, but not all of them were ultimately successful:

WE WANTED TO accomplish the ability to stay in this community, stay with the poorest of the residents, and offer healthcare services and at the same time be financially secure and prepare to offer the continuum of services that would be needed and that we didn't have at the time.   [board chair, financially struggling merger]

OUR MISSION IS healthcare for everyone, not just the poor. We want to satisfy the health needs of everyone, and we felt that by having the suburban and city campuses together and not competing, we could do that.   [board chair, eventual failed merger]

WE NEEDED TO show everybody that we could work together and have a common goal, and that we could accomplish that goal better together than we could separately.
                                [board chair, successful merger]

OUR GOAL WAS to eliminate the competition between the two hospitals, to take advantage of the limited resources that are left to support hospitals in our area, and to keep out the larger city hospital and anyone else.   [board chair, eventual failed merger]

These two employees had a particularly difficult time accepting the need for mergers at the outset. Eventually, though, they saw the benefits of merger:

SOME OF THE employees had strong feelings that they didn't want the merger to happen. They felt, "That's Hospital X, and this is Hospital Y." But stop and think about how we can serve out there. We don't want the people to drive all the way to the city on that awful Route X to get services we can't provide. If we can't do something here, what's wrong with using Hospital X?

> [employee, successful merger]

OUR PATIENT CAN now come to our partner hospital for their heart problems. Avoiding the big city, I think, is the best thing. Our partner has some services that the patients out here can take advantage of without having to go too far out of their way.

> [employee, successful merger]

This community representative saw the business realities of the merger very clearly, but then had to watch the vision fall apart at a later point:

DEREGULATION MEANT THE insurers were free to negotiate whatever rates they wanted, so they could play one hospital against the other or one system against another. Hospitals that don't work together can get even more competitive.

> [community representative, eventual failed merger]

A clinic patient who did not want to be interviewed at first because she felt educationally inadequate spoke from her heart about the merger. She showed much more passion about the dealings between the two local hospitals than many other patients, some of whom were unaware or unconcerned:

I WOULD LIKE to see the hospitals continue to operate together— buy things together and give them out together, and exchange ideas and so forth. I just don't want to see them be shut down. God knows we need them.   [patient, eventual failed merger]

Overcoming competition and working together, then, is a merger expectation not only in the successful mergers but also in the ones that were less successful. Goodness of purpose cannot be underestimated, nor can the forging of trust among players be taken for granted. Setting aside decades of competition on behalf of what is best for a community truly takes big organizations— and big leaders.

SURVIVE, CONTINUE IN THE MISSION, DECREASE
COSTS, GAIN MARKET SHARE

Hospitals in financial distress spend considerable time and effort to remedy that bleak situation. Hospitals that are not in financial distress look at their operations, as well as at future trends, and take steps to remain solvent. No matter what the financial situation, hospitals use every opportunity to maintain and enhance their mission. In some cases, a merger provides the best prospect for survival, preserving the mission, and growing.

Premerger expectations of cost efficiencies may be only partly accurate after a merger. Projected cost savings are often easier to calculate than to actualize. Circumstances may not fit the ideal, the situation may not go as planned, or goals may simply take longer than expected to achieve. Nevertheless, a common thread in merger planning—whether successful or unsuccessful in the end—is the hope that the merger will effect cost savings between the joining partners.

Executives had strong views on what the merger meant to their hospitals' ability to survive and continue their missions. In the following statements, try to pick out which mergers show the most promise:

WE UNDERTOOK THE merger to remain financially solvent and also to maintain the mission of serving the poor in the inner city area—to make sure there was an emergency room for urgent services. We also wanted to make sure the services in the suburbs were maintained. To serve the Medicaid population, you need to have paying customers as well. If you don't have that balance, you're going to end up going down the tubes.

[executive, eventual failed merger]

WHAT REALLY DROVE us was positioning ourself in a market where we had enough of an area and a presence that people couldn't leverage us against our neighbors. That is, quite frankly, what was being done.   [executive, successful merger]

WE DIDN'T GO into this merger to reduce our costs. We didn't go into it to consolidate services per se, because we'd be compromising our mission to make sure that healthcare was available locally. We're very much committed to community-based healthcare, and we are trying to "circle the wagons" to ensure our own survival.

[CEO, successful merger]

SOME PEOPLE WOULD consolidate solely for the cost efficiency— consolidation can reduce costs. That's not why we did it. We look at cost efficiency and we say, "That's a benefit, but that's not really why we consolidated. We did it so we could grow market share, because we wanted to become indispensable to the marketplace."

[executive, successful merger]

THROUGH THE AFFILIATION, we have taken a good number of beds out of the local community system, and we've gotten a lot of very positive comments.   [executive, financially struggling merger]

WE THOUGHT WE could save some money through the consolidation, but savings was not a driving force.

[executive, successful merger]

THE MERGER WILL put in place an appropriate delivery system for the market that is cost effective. It also will make sure that this market is served.   [executive, financially struggling merger]

All the board chairs acted as true leaders of their boards. They have the scars to prove it, but they gained many kudos for having had the courage to preserve and promote their hospitals' missions:

> OUR GOAL WAS to have a single signature authority to deal with insurers so that we could remain independent of tertiary facilities. And we could be a sort of neutral party playing with all the players and attempt to guarantee that those who were accustomed to using a particular doctor and a particular hospital could continue to do that. We didn't want to be just a transport center for the tertiary hospitals in the city.   [board chair, successful merger]

> SOME OF THE industrial people sit on our boards, and we were always asking for their input. It was obvious to us that they wanted cheaper healthcare. We could provide cheaper healthcare by combining efforts, and they've had a lot of input in our doing that. If by joining forces we could do more with less than we were currently doing, the ultimate outcome would be cheaper operations for the employers.   [board chair, successful merger]

> ONE OF THE ideas that came out of the merger was that because we were not going to need all the space for inpatient care, we would try to incorporate nursing home space to save money.
> [board chair, eventual failed merger]

> OUR HOSPITAL WAS much higher on the learning curve, in my opinion, than the board here was. So we were trying to convince them. Their basic the attitude was, "We're fine; why should we bother with this affiliation?" We were trying to say, "You won't be fine in two years. You won't be fine in three years. The community—not just the hospitals—will suffer. Everybody is involved here."
> [board chair, eventual failed merger]

One optimistic physician stayed above the contentious debates to offer this thought on the relationship of financial stability and achieving the mission:

I SEE TWO goals: financial stability and stability of services. By joining together, there is a better likelihood that the financial situation can improve and grow stronger, and that would then allow the services to strengthen and expand.

[physician, financially struggling merger]

A community representative expressed financial expectations of a merger and pointed out that different groups expect different merger results:

OF COURSE THERE is no community; there are subsections within the community. For example, the people in the industrial management group have the perception that they're going to get some bottom-line savings due to the merger.

[long-term care administrator, financially struggling merger]

Similarly, employees vary in their expectations of a merger. Employees were not only well informed about healthcare trends in general but also were knowledgeable about the dynamics of their particular mergers. Each employee has a viewpoint; hospitals might benefit by analyzing employee expectations and perceptions:

WE KNEW WE'D get eaten up if we didn't start working together. The bigger companies were all around the borders. And what a prime opportunity we were—two little sitting ducks up here.

[employee, successful merger]

A HOSPITAL WANTS to serve its patients the best way it can. It also has to be on top of things to get its bills paid and to get the insurance companies to pay. Patient care is the priority, as well as money. We have to get the money to have a place to treat the patients.

[employee, financially struggling merger]

BASICALLY, WE WATCHED them close the other hospital. It was a hospital of our size, and they closed it. We didn't want that for our community. We've been here forever, and we want to stay here and take care of the community. That's why we began merger talks.

[employee, successful merger]

BY JOINING TOGETHER, at least we can survive and be in that five-year plan. And no matter where healthcare takes us, we can grow and do it together. We now have the bigness we needed— we're not too small. We're just right, so we can move on. The merger has taken the scary part away. That helps.

[employee, successful merger]

IN A FEW years there will probably be a lot of new employees sitting around complaining about the older employees who are still talking about the good old days. I'm just glad that the merger came, because I would hate to see either one of these hospitals close. I grew up here, and I do have feelings for my city.

[employee, eventual failed merger]

Achieving savings and decreased costs of operations through merger requires a host of factors to be in alignment. A merger plays out each day, around the clock, in the care that is rendered by the now-joined hospitals. The financial performance depends on all the other factors in the net of meshed missions, philosophies, policies, and procedures; cooperative employee movement between the campuses; physician support and utilization; and community perception and reaction.

The mission is a sacred trust. Also sacred is the responsibility to keep the hospital's doors open on behalf of a community that expects to receive local community care in perpetuity. The need for survival can make a merger decision seem like the most attractive alternative, but the need for survival alone, as compelling as it is, does not ensure merger success.

The organizations involved in both successful and less-than-successful mergers have clearly outlined expectations. The desired outcomes are similar from hospital to hospital: improved quality, autonomy, collaboration, and survival.

What We Have Heard

Goal	Successful Merger	Less-Than-Successful Merger
Improve quality and expand services	yes	yes
Provide for the community and maintain autonomy	yes	yes
Eliminate competition and work together	yes	yes
Survive, continue in the mission, decrease costs, gain market share	yes	yes

Clues and Hallmarks

Did you detect anything in the comments of people involved in successful mergers that indicates a greater sense of clarity or focus compared with the views of individuals who experienced less-than-successful mergers?

Chapter 4

UNDERSTANDING HOW THE HOSPITALS FIT TOGETHER

DISCOVERING GREATER ALIGNMENT THAN EXPECTED

Before a hospital merger, the potential partners often focus on their differences. After the merger, however, the participants often realize that the two hospitals are remarkably similar. A common, pleasant conclusion is that fundamentally, hospital missions really involve just one thing: taking care of other people. Although particular approaches to carrying out the missions certainly vary amid legacies of founding fathers and philosophical underpinnings, mergers uncover a world of similarities between the partners.

The following physicians, who had privileges at both merging hospitals, agree that even apparently dissimilar hospitals can turn out to be remarkably alike:

MY EXPERIENCE INCLUDES many years of very active service at both hospitals. Both had, and continue to have, providers—nurses, staff, and so on—who are equally sincere, dedicated, and concerned for patient needs and patient welfare. And both have had a mission of concern for the poor; that part is definitely the same.
[physician, eventual failed merger]

THE RELATIONSHIP BETWEEN Hospital X in this city and its current partner, Hospital Y, in a nearby city, has always been adversarial. If

somebody would have told us six years ago that we would be working together, everybody would have laughed. There was a competitive, we're-better-than-you attitude on both sides. Neither side wanted anything to do with the other. The merger took probably two years of meetings where each side found out the other guys didn't have three eyes and horns. Each side started to find out that the other side was human, and then we could negotiate an alliance.
[physician, successful merger]

I WORKED IN both hospitals, and I thought there was very little difference.   [physician, financially struggling merger]

Even board chairs, who spend much more time out in the community analyzing perceptions than they do inside the hospitals themselves, saw a great degree of alignment between merging hospitals:

THE HOSPITALS ARE very, very similar. Our hospital is a lot smaller, but the hospitals have similar kinds of people who are most active on their medical staffs. If the core people from both hospitals were compared, very similar kinds of people would be found in each group.   [board chair, successful merger]

OUR MISSIONS WERE pretty much the same except that ours didn't have words specific to one religious denomination in it.
[board chair, eventual failed merger]

Community representatives also saw a high degree of similarity between the two merging hospitals. Whether the two hospitals were known to be long-time rivals or had a more collaborative relationship, a deep-down similarity was noted:

OF COURSE, THERE is the issue of Hospital X's being a hospital of a specific denomination. But the partner hospital, I think, has always been a Christian organization with attention to the poor. In a sense, there's a lot more homogeneity than one might have expected.

        [community representative, financially struggling merger]

IF YOU LOOKED at the missions of both hospitals before they came together, there was certainly some overlap. That's what made the alliance a little bit easier to achieve. Both hospitals were very committed to the communities around them. Both were very committed to quality service, and then they varied in how they delivered that.

        [community representative, financially struggling merger]

Executives echoed the sentiments already expressed—with the exception of one human resources executive. Perhaps because she was immersed in culture issues and was in close touch with employees, she expressed a difference between the two hospitals in terms of their differing sizes. Her comment appears first, followed by those of other executives:

MY PERCEPTION FROM human resources at our hospital was that we had much more caring, loving service providers. They were much more attentive to the needs of patients and to each other. But when we came over to be part of the partner hospital, I found that the competencies of the people there—the caring—were just as strong as at our hospital. The difference, I would say, is the size of the organization. Our hospital is roughly half the size of our partner hospital. At the smaller place, the service providers were much closer, because they worked more closely together. There were fewer of them, so to speak, so they spent more time with one another— there were fewer on a shift. That aspect would be the only difference I see.   [executive, successful merger]

THE PERCEPTION WAS that in terms of culture and values, there were major gaps between the merging hospitals. I think that perception has been fueled by the competitive nature of their systems.

As they have been brought together, the organizations have come to realize that they were a lot more aligned than they ever envisioned. But as with every situation, there are skeletons in the closet. There are cultural issues that have been there, and historical issues. What we've tried to do is recognize those issues as they've existed, and examine which aspects we should try to maintain so that the employees can have some anchoring.   [CEO, successful merger]

THIS IMMEDIATE AREA is very blue-collar oriented. Our partner hospital's city, on the other hand, is pretty affluent. I think that a lot of people in the community thought the consolidation would never work because of that difference. But what's interesting is that we have a lot of people who work at the partner hospital and live here, and vice versa. It's not as different as a lot of people thought it would be.   [executive, successful merger]

BEFORE THE MERGER I would have said, "You need to go to Hospital X, because they're a much more caring and closer group. But I've found that the care at Hospital Y is just as good; the people here care just as much. It's a cultural perception; people are still living with blinders on and don't want to accept the fact that people at Hospital Y care as much as they do at Hospital X.
                    [executive, successful merger]

THE OTHER HOSPITAL was afraid of us; when we'd expand our OR, they would want to do the same thing. There were more similarities than I think people were willing to allow themselves to acknowledge. But after we got into the confidentiality statements and so on, the board started looking under the sheets, so to speak, and found a lot of similarity.   [executive, successful merger]

HOSPITAL X IS a larger organization, but now that I work there, I still see that friendliness among the people. That was one of my major concerns when my office moved from Hospital Y to over here. How would I fit in? But I found a friendly atmosphere. I was really pleased. I was concerned at first, because before, there was a we-versus-they mentality. The two hospitals were so close—there are only 4 miles between us. And it was a competitive atmosphere. I think Hospital X looked at itself as being excellent, whereas it felt we were not. We looked at ourselves as being excellent, but that they were not.   [executive, successful merger]

AFTER BEING IN both the partner hospitals, I'd say that people are people. There's not any major difference in the people. I had heard rumors that they were awful over here, and I got over here and the people are wonderful! The old mentality, the old competitiveness, was still there in the mind-set. But they're good people in both places.   [executive, successful merger]

Two employees who had been forced to shift their work sites because of the merger changes were among the most qualified to speak about alignment. They directly experienced it from the time they began going to work every day at the "other hospital." Alignment was indeed the hallmark:

THE THING I'VE been pleased about since I've gone over to the partner hospital is that the staff people are very, very helpful and friendly. The image that they have around here is that the hospital is in an elite community, a rich town. Well, the people who work there are just plain, ordinary folks trying to do their jobs, just like the people here.   [employee, successful merger]

IT'S AMAZING THAT people actually think that just because you work at another building in another part of town, you're a different kind of person. People really are the same to me, anywhere.
                    [employee, eventual failed merger]

A final comment from a patient who had received services in both hospitals before the merger offers a philosophical slant on public perception of alignment:

> I KNOW PEOPLE who have been in both hospitals who have been really, really satisfied. It depends on how you think about something and how you feel, or on what your experiences have been.
>
> [patient, eventual failed merger]

Being able to overcome long-ingrained competition starts with the realization that people in merging entities are not very different at all. Most everyone is out to do a good job. In hospitals, that good job is done on behalf of other persons, which takes physicians and staff who care and who also project this caring attitude to the patients and the public. Doing a good job is a universal underpinning that goes beyond any one hospital's walls.

DISCOVERING GREATER DIFFERENCES THAN EXPECTED

Most hospitals have striking similarities, but even successful mergers can discover the opposite: "We knew the merging hospitals were different, but we never dreamed just how different they really were." Although this realization might not derail a merger, it presents an ongoing challenge to merger leaders to craft an organization that will be strong enough to withstand the forces continuing to pull the partners apart.

This topic will be analyzed here by hospital executives only. Walking into a newly merged organization creates a personal struggle for any executive, whether he or she was a part of one of the premerger hospitals or was recruited from outside the organization to be part of the merged entity.

One CEO spoke about the physicians and the need for sensitivity of timing in bringing the two groups together:

I THINK DOCS are different culturally. The medical staffs are different. I think it was the right decision not to consolidate medical staffs; such a marriage would have been tough for us. We're going to let that sort of work its way through over time—no rush on that.

[CEO, successful merger]

Overcoming past cultures in each hospital is a very real challenge after a merger. Over the many years that each hospital has been in existence, individual organizational cultures have been created, nurtured, and experienced. This makes the postmerger unifying process more challenging:

THE HOSPITALS ARE different—very different—almost like night and day. I think the former administration at Hospital X put the fear of God into people and they basically operated under fear. The people there were always covering themselves, whatever they did, and they were always competing and had a whole different way. Here at Hospital Y there was more of a team approach. The managers didn't feel threatened, and I think that filtered down to the employees. It just seems very different.

[executive, eventual failed merger]

THE TWO ORGANIZATIONS are very different—more different than my past experiences would have indicated. This hospital was much more diverse, much more extreme. And I'm not sure anyone really appreciated that difference. Not only was it not appreciated; I don't think it was even thought to be an issue that would interfere with the organization.

[CEO, eventual failed merger]

THE CULTURES OF the two towns are different; the cultures of the communities are different; the cultures of the hospitals are different. They are more different than I thought."

[executive, successful merger]

A major area to be addressed in a merger, from the employees' standpoint, is benefits and other personnel administration issues. This human resources executive was exasperated at what she faced in trying to bring the two hospitals together:

THERE WERE VERY different approaches to negotiating styles. At one of our campuses, the part-timers were basically lower than life. At the other campus, they were recognized as being very valuable, because for every full-timer in a 14-day schedule there was a part-timer, so this person was really critical to the success of the organization. That was a philosophical difference between the campuses.
[executive, successful merger]

Another CEO was extremely frustrated with the obstacles he encountered almost every step of the way in getting his merger launched. The financial problems were not going away easily, but that was just one of the challenges brought on by basic differences between hospitals in the merger, which struggled then and continues to struggle today.

MEDICAL STAFFS WERE different. One was a teaching hospital and the other a nonteaching hospital. The boards were different. Hospital X had a much more community-focused board, while at Hospital Y much more authority nested with the sponsors, and the system did not give the board full power. Management styles and ways of doing things were a lot different. Just walking around, one could see that the cultures at the two facilities were different.
[CEO, financially struggling merger]

FOR ALL THE cultural compatibility, the pace is different at the two organizations, and that has been problematic in a number of areas. It was something I recognized up front and something we have to deal with, but the pace and the expectations around pace are very different. One hospital feels that "God will provide," whereas the other hospital says, "We've got to do this; we've got to get it done." There are constant clashes.

[executive, financially struggling merger]

Perhaps one of the more amazing phenomena of merger dynamics is that despite differences between the partners, a successful outcome can be forged. The strength to keep the merger solid comes from somewhere to avoid self-destruction; that strength is really in the leaders who stay focused on the end result and can navigate through the ostensible differences.

BUILDING TRUST, CONSIDERING CULTURE, AND OVERCOMING PAST GRIEVANCES

Whether or not the partnering hospitals are more aligned or less aligned than expected, the postmerger challenge is to create a new organization out of two former entities. Cultures are entrenched. Philosophies are long-standing. There is plenty of "Styrofoam in the landfill"—those things that can be unearthed in a million years and still not have biodegraded but look as fresh as they did when they were placed there, much like past human hurts and slights.

People have long memories. Any breach of trust is not easily forgotten but remains with us as the yardstick by which we measure faithfulness. Organizations are merely an aggregate of people with those long memories—the very people who have a lot to overcome when two entities merge. One community representative expresses this idea from a fundamental root-cause perspective:

I THINK THAT the two cities where the two hospitals are located are still arguing about who's going to be the county seat, as they've argued for the past hundred years.

[community representative, successful merger]

One of the nurses from a successful merger was very supportive of the merger itself, because she and a counterpart at the other
hospital had been collaborating for many years. She commented
on the lack of trust between the two hospitals with a marked
sadness in her voice:

> THERE WAS NO communication between the hospitals. The other
> nurse and I shared the most data. It was out of mutual respect, just
> us two, but my peers here would say, "Why do you talk to her? What
> do you tell her? You can't tell her that! What is she going to do?"
> The two hospitals have been rivals—big-time rivals—for many,
> many, many years.   [employee, successful merger]

Competition was keenly expressed in discussions of medical
staff matters. Physicians easily become entrenched in the com-
forts and mores of the hospitals they like to use. Those physicians
who are not subject to steerage of patients generally gravitate to
the hospital they prefer, for whatever reason. Change of the magnitude that is created by a merger understandably has far-reaching
tremors:

> THE MEDICAL STAFF at one of the two hospitals came into this
> merger feeling pretty skeptical, so we really had to build up trust,
> which we spent a lot of time doing. The medical staff at that hospi-
> tal functions as a whole. They have a couple committees. I don't
> know the history, but they don't trust each other very much. They
> insist on being in a room together before reaching consensus. They
> won't appoint representatives, because that's not how they func-
> tion. For years they have worked through executive medical leader-
> ship, and they have trusted that group in the process, so it's been a
> real journey from that standpoint.   [CEO, successful merger]

> WE PHYSICIANS GOT together—about eight of us—over the
> two-year period, and we were just getting used to one another. The

physicians from the other hospital wanted to maintain their identity. The doctors here were feeling, "I don't want to have to go over to that hospital and work; I want to stay here." They didn't say it exactly, but they felt that this hospital was bigger and better, and they didn't want to have to step down to the other hospital. And the other hospital didn't want to lose its identity.

[physician, successful merger]

BEFORE THE AFFILIATION, it was a nice, confined, dedicated war between the two hospitals. The CEOs, on the surface, shook each other's hands, smiled at meetings, and things like that. Unfortunately, behind closed doors, although they didn't hate each other personally, they hated the institution that the other stood for because it meant competition. [physician, eventual failed merger]

THE CULTURES AT the two hospitals are very, very different. Hospital X tends to want to be isolationist and special, because they're in a richer neighborhood; they have that attitude. Unfortunately, they were getting eaten alive by the people downtown. They came to a sobering thought: "We can't do this anymore; we're not surviving doing this." They came to that realization begrudgingly, and they still come to it begrudgingly. [physician, successful merger]

THE DOCTORS DO not like clinical consolidation, and the health system does mean that. Unfortunately, they're going to continue to fight it, although we're doing everything we can to bring them together. [physician, eventual failed merger]

Culture is a prized possession of any organization. It is especially important to hospitals, because the services they provide are very labor intensive. Although hospitals use a variety of equipment and technology, the usefulness of it depends on the human beings who operate it and interpret the results. Culture, although appreciated, is also a stumbling block when people must move forward:

I WASN'T HERE before the merger, but a lot of old perspectives held on even postmerger. People were having difficulty adjusting from the "them and us" to the "us and us" mentality. That problem held on for a while, but we're finally getting past most of it.

[employee, successful merger]

CULTURALLY, WE WERE dealing with a religious-denomination hospital and a nondenominational hospital. We discussed that early on. We knew that was a challenge. And the denomination-nondenomination difference was sometimes used as an excuse for an argument. It really came down to people—and I don't blame them—being very protective of their jobs, what they did, and where they wanted to go.   [board chair, eventual failed merger]

HOSPITAL X HAD a very strong culture. One of its distinguishing characteristics was stability, both in the employee ranks and in the management ranks. Another characteristic that stood out, certainly, was having a CEO who was there for many years. So the hospital had a stable, very paternalistic kind of culture related to its employees. It was almost a sleepy culture. Even though it was part of a turbulent healthcare market, the hospital was kind of an oasis of stability for many, many years. And to some extent, it makes the coming together more difficult, because many people have been at Hospital X a long time.

[executive, successful merger]

HOSPITAL X HAS a reputation of being much more laid back, and Hospital Y is much more type A in terms of staff behavior. From the Hospital X perspective, the Hospital Y people tend to be not caring, more business oriented, and all of that. From the Hospital Y perspective, Hospital X does not pay attention to the business aspects of things; perhaps people are lazy. From a cultural perspective, this has caused some struggles.

[community representative, financially struggling merger]

A man who had lived in the community for years had dealt with both merging hospitals and was a trusted authority about the two organizations. He agreed that culture can hinder mergers:

> THE EMPLOYEES WHO originated from Hospital X would have pride in their quality service and their business expertise. If you talked to employees who originated from Hospital Y, they would tell you that their hospital is a family, and it has heart. Now that's true in both cases, but the two hospitals see each other as being very different.
>
> [community representative, financially struggling merger]

As the preceding comments reveal, successful mergers are not any different than less successful mergers in ease of bringing the organizations together. Challenges abound for every hospital when the task is such a daunting one—that is, taking two previous competitors and making them into one cohesive, functioning unit. Successful mergers, however, are able to meet that daunting challenge and go beyond it, achieving the prized oneness that is the merger's purpose. Even though the Styrofoam may still be there when the merger is unearthed in a million years, it has been contained, isolated, understood, and passed over.

COMPARING PARTNERS FINANCIALLY PREMERGER

Any number of consultants can make a premerger comparison of partnering hospitals using a variety of indexes, but the prevalent interest is always finances. Are both hospitals solvent? How much debt does each one carry? What is the patient mix at each, and what are the future prospects for handling a combined market share based on that patient mix?

Negative results of such financial probing require a thorough assessment of the potential risks in attaining financial viability after the merger.

The following people who offered comments can be grouped into two camps: those persons who felt that each merging hospital was doing well financially and those who felt that each merging hospital was not doing well financially. Note the correlation between hospital solvency and the merger outcome:

IN REGARD TO profits and losses, both hospitals stacked up pretty well. The other hospital probably was more stable financially. We had some good, profitable years when I came, but both hospitals were pretty consistent. On the balance sheet, we were both strong. We're two of the lower-cost providers in the region according to cost per adjusted discharge. We were not a burden to each other in that regard.   [CEO, successful merger]

I'VE ALWAYS UNDERSTOOD that both hospitals have been rather solvent. From the word on the street, I don't think there were major problems like there were at that nearby small hospital back then. Those problems were well known to everybody.
                    [community representative, successful merger]

THERE WAS A time when Hospital X's financial outlook was kind of ominous. It was having financial problems, and it primarily related to leadership. Then the leadership changed, and it got back on track and started toward an improved financial picture. A while ago, Hospital Y was in a pretty bad financial shape. It had a lot of problems with cost reports, receivables. During this period of time we took it from a relatively weak organization to a considerably stronger one financially. At the time of the affiliation, I think both hospitals were reasonably strong financially.
                    [executive, successful merger]

ONCE THE TWO hospitals got into discussion and negotiation, it was looking like both were financially sound, so there were a lot of similarities. We were headed toward the same financial goals—cost per discharge and things like that—so we were both looking in the same direction.   [executive, successful merger]

EVEN THOUGH HOSPITAL X was larger, when you looked at the balance sheets of the two organizations, you realized that quite frankly, they were very similar. The equity in them was not that different, because Hospital Y had less debt, and Hospital X had a little more. So we looked at everything and said, "Let's go in as equals." And that's basically what happened.

[executive, successful merger]

Merger success is less likely when the partners are each struggling with finances:

BOTH OUR HOSPITALS HAD historically been on the cusp of being profitable/nonprofitable and had years of floating back and forth. We each had different focuses but financially had performed marginally; we never created big cash reserves. Hospital X, our hospital, has had the ability to fall back on the sponsor's financial strength to do a variety of different things that it could not do alone. And Hospital Y tried to make individual entities self-sustaining from a financial perspective. We were able to pull cash and use cash from the hospital as seed money—working capital for some of the organizations as they grew.   [executive, financially struggling merger]

HOSPITAL X WAS not making money—let's put it that way. I think Hospital Y was also on the edge. No hospital in town was making money. In this state, very few hospitals make money.

[physician, financially struggling merger]

I THINK THE situation was that we had to go to a full merger of operations as quickly as possible. Individually, neither institution had the financial strength to just sit around for the next two to five years to see how it would go."

[executive, financially struggling merger]

I THINK BOTH hospitals can claim by their balance sheets that they are losing money. On the bottom line, they are losing money.

[community representative, eventual failed merger]

HOSPITAL X WAS losing too much money. It couldn't afford to keep losing money. In fact, both hospitals were losing. Hospital Y would have had to merge with some other hospital; it could not have stood on its own.   [trustee, eventual failed merger]

One community representative's sentiments provided an accurate overview of the situation in his community. It was ironic, however, that the hospital merger in that community could not keep itself together.

WITHOUT THE MERGER, I don't think there would have been a Hospital X before too long. I know that both hospitals are having trouble.   [community representative, eventual failed merger]

An analysis of the collected comments seems to suggest that hospitals that are solvent when they merge create a new entity that remains solvent, whereas hospitals that are in financial distress when they merge cannot count on the merger to save their financial situation. This generalization needs to be tested. Meanwhile, one losing hospital plus one losing hospital seems to equal all the market share, but all the financial problems as well.

ACHIEVING FINANCIAL STRENGTH FROM THE MERGER

The hospitals studied that experienced successful mergers were able to quantify a marked financial strength that was attributed directly to the merger. They also embodied the merger goals and expectations outlined earlier: survival, expanding services, improving quality of care, avoiding duplication, and realizing cost efficiencies. If a merger does not result in financial strength, however, fulfilling any of the other merger expectations becomes almost impossible.

Achieving postmerger financial strength is a testament to concerted premerger planning and philosophical meshing:

> WE'VE ACCOMPLISHED ONE thing together: the financial structure of this organization. The two hospitals and physicians together are much stronger than each is alone. [executive, successful merger]

Capitalists fully understand the power of cash in the bank: it creates a vista of opportunity limited only by how far the money will go. The following executives noted that fact:

> ONE OF THE big reasons for forming the merger is financial. I wouldn't say it's the number one goal, but in healthcare you always have to be thinking about the financials—and that has definitely paid off. The organizations as a whole are more profitable than they've ever been, because most of the savings are coming from back-room expenses. We have joint purchasing agreements now and things like that. In management, one person is now doing what two people used to do. Those sorts of savings are there.
>
> [executive, successful merger]

> THERE HAVE BEEN so many positives. The financial aspect always seems to be one measure. Financially, the merger and each of the entities are a lot stronger than they were individually. Healthy margins have been created. [CEO, successful merger]

> WE JUST REISSUED all of our bonds, and we got two bumps from the rating agency, up to an AA–, which in today's world is really amazing. The rating agency looked at us financially and also looked at

where we were going—the direction and our plans to get there. To me, that indicated that the merger, at least from an outside perspective, was the right thing to do.   [executive, successful merger]

The employees in one merger were skeptical about the true motivations of their hospitals merging. The staff had a nagging fear that the merger had occurred to make it easier to close one of the hospitals. An executive summarized his response:

WE'RE INVESTING LARGE sums of money for renovation and remodeling. It's giving the employees some feeling of security to know that we wouldn't be spending $2 million on a med/surg unit if were going to close it tomorrow.   [executive, successful merger]

Finally, one of the proudest persons interviewed was a board chair who felt that the merger had been well worth undertaking because of the numerous strategic improvements that resulted:

WE THINK THAT we're in a mode right now where we can dictate to another organization, such as a health system or a bigger hospital, because we've done something that everybody has watched and applauded us for doing. A good example is that we have a physician hospital organization. When some of the insurance companies tried to short-stop that process, they found out that they couldn't climb all the way over the wall, because our alliance was strong enough and everybody hung together. I think that's something that other hospitals and health systems are looking at.

[board chair, successful merger]

EXPERIENCING FINANCIAL WEAKNESS FROM THE MERGER

Just as successful mergers are characterized by postmerger financial strength, mergers that would judge themselves to be less than successful have the common characteristic of disappointing postmerger financial performance. Financial results can be compromised despite the most well-motivated merger goals because of factors such as insufficient premerger planning, unanticipated changes in market conditions, or acceleration of the merger process.

One CEO expressed the depths of his personal struggle about where his merger needed to go next. I vividly recall the quiet, almost inaudible way he expressed himself:

> THERE'S A VERY limited series of choices. Either we find a way to solve the financial problems, or we take the whole thing apart. And if we take it apart, I think we will have gone way too far for this hospital to magically reopen. It would take an act of God for the doctors to come back here, plus the staff and everything else. And taking it apart is likely to require more cash. So if we're going to go forward, what does that mean? Is the commitment there? What cash is required to get there? And what about the mortgage?
>
> [CEO, financially struggling merger]

Other comments note the disappointment that was felt about the postmerger financial situation:

> WE HAD HOPED to be able to refinance debt across the system through an obligated group kind of arrangement that would save us over $1 million in interest costs. We have not been able to do that.   [executive, financially struggling merger]

> THE BOTTOM FELL out of our volume and we lost millions last year and millions this year—probably we'll lose millions next year. We never anticipated numbers like that, so no one said, "OK, if that happens, where will the cash come from?
>
> [CEO, financially struggling merger]

Internal operational challenges of merger can exacerbate the downward spiral:

WE'RE HAVING GREAT difficulty finding the right numbers of people to cut. Staffing in this state tends to be a lot lower on a full-time basis, so the opportunities aren't there.

[executive, financially struggling merger]

A LOT OF things have changed since day one. The community's more competitive, the volume has dropped, and rates are higher. There was a huge assumption about expenses that didn't come true. Again, we deal with what we have to. We take our best guess and try.   [CEO, financially struggling merger]

Despite financial problems, one board chair continued to believe that a merger was in the best interest of everyone in the community. This comment foreshadows other problems that would follow and ultimately be responsible for the demise of the merger:

As WE WENT forward, the economic situation looked more and more dire. There was almost ... I don't want to say a panic. There was a real acceleration in implementing this plan, in coming up with a clinical consolidation.

[board chair, eventual failed merger]

The scenes portrayed by these voices are very different from the ones generated by the previous descriptions of financially successful mergers. The players in failed or struggling mergers would stress the need to pay attention to conscientious premerger planning, due diligence, and creating a contingency strategy.

Both successful and unsuccessful mergers can have an alignment of culture, operations, and procedures. These characteristics are crucial, but they are only part of the ingredients for success. Postmerger financial strength arose in the interviews time after time as the one characteristic necessary to enable organizations to meet their merger goals and expectations. Is it possible that hospitals, which have care missions, must ultimately succumb to the overarching domination of finances?

What We Have Heard

	Successful Merger	Less-Than-Successful Merger
Discovering greater alignment than expected	yes	yes
Discovering greater differences than expected	yes	yes
Building trust, considering culture, and overcoming past grievances	yes	yes
Comparing partners financially premerger	yes	yes
Achieving financial strength from the merger	yes	no
Experiencing financial weakness from the merger	no	yes

Clues and Hallmarks

Did you detect anything in the comments of people involved in successful mergers that indicated a greater sense of fit than was evident in the less-than-successful mergers? Are mergers of financially struggling organizations doomed to financial problems?

Chapter 5

CREATING A GOVERNANCE STRUCTURE

Determining the governance structure for a merged hospital entity is a decision that affects every facet and fiber of the new organization. The board is the ultimate umbrella for oversight, policymaking, and fiduciary accountability. Individual hospitals have boards that perform this function very well. Merged hospitals, however, present a new challenge in handling those same duties. The complexity of the challenge depends on how easily and quickly the existing boards arrive at an acceptable approach to governing the new organization.

Merged hospital entities face many crucial governance decisions: Are the existing hospital boards merely going to join and be retitled as the board for the newly merged entity? Are the existing hospital boards to be eliminated and an entirely new board appointed to govern the merger? Are some sitting trustee positions to be eliminated, no matter what structure is chosen?

The solutions to those problems depend on several factors, including personalities and egos, the leadership skills desired, individuals' commitment to the project and to the community, and the ability to put aside old organizational identities on behalf of the new one.

SUPERBOARD APPROACH

A trustee described one approach—the "superboard" approach—to the creation of a new board for a merger:

> BASICALLY WHAT WE have are the boards for each organization and then this superboard, which is the board for the merger entity. But the assets stay with each community. That was a major decision in bringing the two hospitals together because of the mentality of the two communities.   [trustee, successful merger]

SINGLE BOARD APPROACH

Once a merger occurs it becomes the entity of focus. The appointment of trustees must be rethought. Sometimes the two hospital boards are dissolved and blended into a single board for the merger:

> WHEN WE REFORMATTED the board, the expectation was that a person who came on this new board was saying very clearly and with commitment that his or her commitment was to the system, not to an individual hospital.   [CEO, eventual failed merger]

However, the creation of a new board is not easy in every merger. These trustees were animated as they told me about the difficult decisions they had to make to create new governance for the merged entity:

> WE HAD A major problem. After this public outcry the members of the board themselves began to polarize along the same lines. Hospital X aligned itself with the vocal community and the inner city, and the partner hospital had its own perspective. That's when we realized that having three boards was not going to work. After several months of unsuccessful attempts to try to reconcile the

three boards, we had to dissolve all three boards and appoint a new board for the merger entity.

[board chair, eventual failed merger]

WE DISSOLVED OUR board—everyone resigned. People on all three boards—from the two original hospitals and from the merger entity—resigned. The final board, I believe, is now smaller than it will be eventually. [trustee, eventual failed merger]

WE SAID, LET'S take the board from Hospital X, take the board from Hospital Y, and come up with one new board—one new group of people. There will be one meeting, with the same people. Everyone will be on the same page all at the same time. So we blended the boards, and that's what we are today: a blended board.

[board chair, eventual failed merger]

Another well-informed board member described her merged entity's approach to creating structure for the new corporation. She had been a supportive trustee from the inception of the merger:

ALTHOUGH WE MERGED boards, we did not really merge employees. We have two separate entities, and the employees are still in their hospitals with a few exceptions. For example, dietary people are going back and forth as a kind of pilot. Really, people aren't feeling a major effect, because they're still in their hospitals. They're comfortable. They can still say, "This is the department I work in. They're down there miles away, and that's OK." We did not merge medical staffs. [trustee, successful merger]

MIRROR BOARDS APPROACH

Some mergers find that the concept of "mirror" boards—two hospital boards that convene for the merged entity—is the most workable governance structure. The concept allows for a much more streamlined approach to handling existing hospital corporations:

> WE TOOK THE two hospital boards, and beginning in the summer, we started having board meetings—everybody came to the whole thing. We'd open the Hospital X meeting, close it, open the Hospital Y meeting, close it. I remember it was terribly formal at first. At the second meeting people asked, "Why are we doing this? Why don't we have one agenda and create two sets of minutes? So the mirror board came about. As a result, the Hospital X people have been involved in issues about Hospital Y for two years and vice versa. And they all think they own it all. In reality, it was almost a year until they actually did!   [CEO, financially struggling merger]

> MIRROR BOARDS WORK, and they work very well. They are a way to cut out the we-versus-they kind of process. And a mirror board is a very simple technique if people can get over the fear of doing it the first time. You have to guard against one thing. If there is a big fight in a meeting and one side says, "We want to meet and talk about it ourselves," that will kill the organization. It must be kept in the same room.   [CEO, financially struggling merger]

BOARD DYNAMICS

These executives and trustees offer advice on what they would do differently. In their case, two boards remain but need to consolidate into one. Their words are worth noting, especially because their comments flow out of a merger situation that can be considered successful.

> PROBABLY THE BIGGEST hornet's nest today is actually the board. This is phase 2 in governance—putting together a structure that gets the job done. Originally, everyone gets a board seat, and there

is a huge infrastructure. It also follows a law of diminishing returns; it doesn't work well. So the board developed a set of principles for streamlining governance, making it more decisive, and so on. Where are we now? The board has rolled out those principles; they've rolled out a game plan to begin to implement. Right now there's a sense of turmoil within the board regarding how this is actually going to occur. When the board is downsized, is the existing leadership going to prevail? And will that leadership take on even more of an assertive role with a smaller board?

[CEO, successful merger]

IF I WERE going to do anything differently, I would have taken more time with the board structuring when we put it together so we wouldn't have to deal with it now. I don't think we did it right. We just did it in the expedient way, because if we hadn't done it that way, we probably wouldn't have gotten the deal done at all. Looking back, if we could have sized the board correctly then and had one board, I wouldn't have had the last two years of problems.

[board chair, successful merger]

I THINK THE biggest disappointment in the merger is the partisan line through the board. I think management has come together very, very well. I think the board lags behind, for two reasons: (1) I think they still remember where they came from, and (2) everything's going well, so there's nothing to focus on.

[executive, successful merger]

Finally, a CEO shares some advice and one of his frustrations about the governance function and style adopted from the beginning of his merger:

MAKE SURE THE board is nimble and in sync with management. In our situation, quite frankly, once management got its act together, we're moving faster; it's almost that the board has become a drag on management. And that's their concern—to be with management and able to support and respond.

[CEO, successful merger]

Comparing the governance structures of successful and less-than-successful mergers would require an extensive research project in its own right. How much effect does that structure have on a merger's outcome? Some successful mergers, in fact, do not have efficient governance structures. And although the concept of mirror boards is very workable, in the interviews this governance structure was found in a struggling merger. There is obviously more to merger success than structure and the approaches taken by boards.

What We Have Heard

Governance Structure	Successful Merger	Less-Than-Successful Merger
Superboard	yes	no
Single board	no	yes
Mirror boards	no	yes
Consolidated board in discord	yes	no

Clues and Hallmarks

Does the governance structure adopted postmerger directly affect the merger's chances of being successful? Does governance structure really matter? Or can boards put the responsibility on management to create a successful operation from the joining partners?

Chapter 6

UNDERSTANDING THE POSTMERGER CONDITIONS

COMMUNICATION

Maintaining good communication in any organization, a key duty of management, is always a challenge. Ensuring that everyone within the organization feels adequately informed borders on the impossible. There is always someone who does not attend a meeting, does not read a memo or announcement, or constantly feels outside the channels of communication. Others choose not to listen or not to believe what they hear.

In a merger, the communications challenge increases exponentially. It is a tireless crusade to explain the who, what, when, why, and how of the merger in the first place, and that effort is followed by the untold demands of conveying the message of merger progress and related changes. Again, the audience may or may not be receptive. Perception is reality, as the following voices indicate.

Many interviewees indicated that communication in their organization was actually better after the merger than before, or it was at least as good as always:

WE ARE KEPT very informed today—at staff meetings and right from the top, we hear what's happening.

[employee, successful merger]

67

I THINK THERE were problems before the merger with how things were done, and I think we're just doing a better job of relating to the people, making them a part of the organization, and making them feel like they're important.   [executive, successful merger]

I WOULD SAY that management lets us employees know more of what's going on than they used to. It might take them six months or so, and by that time we've already forgotten what they told us, but at least they've informed us.   [employee, successful merger]

THERE HAVE BEEN many more meetings since the merger. And we now have e-mail and PCs, which we never had before, so we can send out messages quickly to everybody. We have a lot more meetings. I think management wants the employees to be informed and to know what's going on. They don't want us to be insecure, in my opinion.   [employee, financially struggling merger]

THE ADMINISTRATION TRIED to make the merger positive, to have meetings and to open things up. So I think that after the initial change has occurred and everybody has settled in, there won't be much difference.   [employee, successful merger]

Two CEO's shared their perspectives on the challenges of trying to keep pace with communication in a newly merged organization because of the demands for information by so many publics:

WE IN THE administration try to communicate; we try to make weekly nursing rounds. The COO conducts open-line meetings at both campuses every week or every other week. Every six months I go out and do around-the-clock employee meetings that are 14, 15, or 16 sessions over a two-week period, both on campus and off campus. These meetings tend to go over pretty well. And we produce a lot of employee newsletters and things like that. We try to communicate.   [CEO, successful merger]

IN TWO YEARS I've put 45,000 miles on a vehicle between campuses. But I'm not a one-man band, and I can't be everywhere and still provide the strategic vision for the organization. So we began putting together a monthly newsletter of written material. We also thought communication was so critical to the organization that we produced videos that we showed at all campuses around the clock to get out certain messages that we wanted to distribute.

[CEO, successful merger]

One physician agreed that the efforts of management to communicate about the merger were bearing fruit and were appreciated:

THE VAST MAJORITY of physicians have been supportive to varying degrees, but all understand the reasons for the merger. And I think it's a testament to the administration that information was as open as it was. [physician, successful merger]

Of course, some people always feel, "No one ever tells me anything." In any organization there will be people who desire more information. The following comments are from persons in merged hospitals that happened to be struggling entities, but similar comments could come from successful mergers.

I THINK THERE'S a change now at Hospital X, because we were told on Friday that our department would be part of a merger organization. We had no inkling of what was going on. I remember that a long time ago the administrator here used to tell us about changes that were coming a long time before they happened. So I think there was more communication before the merger.

[employee, eventual failed merger]

SINCE THE MERGER, I haven't felt that we employees are always in the know. Though there are informative meetings where we are told, "This is so," or "That is fact," and things are working, the information just doesn't seem accurate all the time.

[employee, eventual failed merger]

THE HOSPITAL STILL keeps us informed. The information doesn't seem as frequent, but the need isn't as great. We have a newsletter that highlights more detail. It comes out once a month, or maybe once a week. I don't usually get a chance to read it—you can see my desk!   [employee, financially struggling merger]

BEFORE THE MERGER, we used to have more meetings, and we were kept informed about things that were going on. We don't seem to have a lot of that anymore. And at the meetings that I have been to, it seemed like when people asked questions the hospital really didn't have the answers or want to give the answers, so people went away unsure. They wondered what was really going on.

[employee, eventual failed merger]

COMMUNICATION WAS BETTER before the merger—not department-wise but just overall. When there was a change, the hospital would have nighttime meetings, and anybody who could come would come. The employees had an opportunity to ask questions. But we really don't have that chance now. The hospital usually just puts something in writing, so communication is not quite as good as it was before.   [employee, eventual failed merger]

It is easy for organizations to write memos, newsletters, and publications telling the story and giving the details. It takes additional effort to check on whether or not those messages are being received. Everyone interviewed who wanted to be supportive of their merger craved information about it. They just wanted to know the truth and the straight story. The additional effort to provide honest information is well spent.

MEDICAL STAFF LINK

The key to every hospital's success is its medical staff. In a community hospital setting, the majority of staff physicians are independent practitioners with no financial ties or formal relationships with the board or administration. A hospital depends on goodwill, good-quality care, good staffing ratios, good employees, and good facilities to give doctors a reason to use the facility rather than take patients to a competitor.

Under times of challenge and the siege of widespread change, as in a merger, that goodwill gets stretched to the limit. Medical staff support for a merger decision and the subsequent clinical aftermath are a function of premerger communication, involvement, and the opportunity to be heard. Physicians place their stakes in a community not only to practice in their profession but also to raise a family and be involved in the fabric of that community—its social networks, school system, churches, housing, shopping, recreation, and so on.

A hospital merger has a great effect on many things in the physicians' community. Physicians have varied reactions, including opinions on how the merging hospitals structure the connection between the respective staffs. Several physicians commented on the early benefits of a merger:

> THERE HAVE BEEN some joint continuing medical education programs. There have also been some joint social events to try to help facilitate communication, understanding, and goodwill among the two staffs. [physician, successful merger]

> WE'VE MERGED THE medical staff offices very quickly. We made all the files available, so that what we called *cross-credentialing* could occur in a short period of time.
> [physician, financially struggling merger]

A PHYSICIAN IS either a Hospital X doctor or a Hospital Y doctor, but the interchange and cooperation is better than it used to be. Now some of the facilities are being extended. For instance, all cardiology from Hospital Y was going to an out-of-town hospital. Just this last year the cardiologists from Hospital X went over to Hospital Y, so it's all one service now.

[physician, successful merger]

Medical staff support for a merger is attained to differing degrees from hospital to hospital. At the same time, the medical staff is a key and essential group whose support or lack of support directly bears on a merger's outcome. The importance of this support was echoed by executives and trustees interviewed. Their comments zeroed in on the synergy resulting from their merged hospitals' medical staffs, which was a tremendous asset in their mergers:

THE BENEFIT WE have always had of this coming together is that it has received a tremendous amount of support from the medical staffs. Beginning to consolidate service ahead of time required lots of communication, but the physicians were ready for it.

[executive, financially struggling merger]

ONCE THE PHYSICIANS saw the boards coming together, they kept saying, "Why are we having two executive committee meetings; why two medical staff meetings?" The physicians reinforced what we were trying to do.   [CEO, financially struggling merger]

THE PHYSICIANS WERE the easiest part of the merger, which was very surprising. Some of the other hospitals had had problems. But most of our physicians were cross-credentialed already and knew the sites.   [board chair, financially struggling merger]

How connected should the medical staffs be when a merger occurs? Two CEOS offer differing views, based on their particular situations:

WE NOW HAVE a single set of medical staff bylaws that has been adopted on both campuses. We now have one central credentialing process, but campus-specific privileges.

[CEO, successful merger]

WE KEPT THE medical staffs separate. Each campus has its own organized medical staff. We did not bring them together.

[CEO, successful merger]

In an ideal world, doctors on medical staffs everywhere would support the idea of a hospital merger in their communities as being in the best interests of those communities. The real world, however, has doctors who are not only clinicians but also human beings who have marked feelings for their communities and their hospitals. Doctors can make or break a hospital merger due to their influential and respected opinions, as well as their ability to "vote with their feet":

THE MEDICAL STAFF was in support of this merger. Were they absolutely happy about it? No. Wouldn't everyone rather stay in their own comfortable situation? I think most people would say yes. But at least the physicians understood everything and for the most part have been willing and committed to going forward with the process.   [physician, financially struggling merger]

THE DOCTORS DO not like clinical consolidation and the health system merger does mean that. Unfortunately, the doctors are going to continue to fight consolidation, although we're doing everything we can to bring them together.   [physician, eventual failed merger]

This frustrated RN spoke for many people in her department as she analyzed her facility's medical staff:

THE DOCTORS HAVE come in and stirred up all kinds of trouble. Maybe they're putting their own feelings into what they want, so they come in and get us going. They'll say things that make us really angry. So now we just kind of listen. We've gotten very mature toward them now. We just listen and say "uh-huh."

[employee, eventual failed merger]

Taking a path of least resistance makes the work day easier to get through. And when hospital workdays are filled with escalating change, no one wants to create more upheaval.

The desired partnership between a hospital and its medical staff must begin with efforts at untiring and dauntless communication between those leaders and physicians to ensure a unified message. And when the message content is about a merger, those communication efforts must now be redoubled.

DEPARTMENT CONSOLIDATIONS

No decisions related to mergers are easily made. Decisions to consolidate departments between two merging hospitals to achieve operational efficiencies and cost savings are likewise difficult. However, a possibly dispassionate decision made in a sequestered boardroom must then be lived out by all who are affected.

The routines of employees and managers are disrupted by consolidation. People must now work shoulder to shoulder with employees of the "other" hospital—people who were the target of competition over the years. Adaptation and tolerance are needed because the daily procedures from two different facilities are examined and fused. The decision to consolidate services may be one of the first "easy" decisions made by the merger leaders, but it changes the complexion of operations from that point on as the ramifications are felt throughout the organization.

The following voices come from people in merged entities that started off with particular departmental consolidations:

WE'VE COMBINED A number of clinical services. We've combined just about all of the support services now. We are at a corporate level for support services, and we are achieving considerable efficiencies as a result.   [executive, successful merger]

THERE HAS BEEN some consolidation—not of the housekeeping but of the laundry, the printing, and some of the ancillary services—that theoretically could reduce some costs. It's good for all of us, obviously, if we can reduce overhead by merging. That would be worthwhile in and of itself.   [physician, successful merger]

THE CEO HAS done a lot, with one director for physical therapy and one director for the operating room. We're now getting ready to go to one director for the nursing department, one for facilities management, and one for dietary/nutrition services. So many of the departments have consolidated into one director, who goes back and forth.   [trustee, successful merger]

WE'VE CONSOLIDATED THE psychiatric services at one of the hospitals, and that has been an effort. We have consolidated pharmacy services, laboratory services—again, for a large part, it is the support services that we have consolidated. We have refined our emergency room coverage to have one medical group at all campuses.   [executive, successful merger]

Staff positions are an easy target for early consolidations, because certain functions can be provided to two sites by one person:

WE HAVE ONE person who's in charge of planning for both institutions. We have one strategic planning committee for both institutions. Our quality management person is now in the process of developing case management protocols and the like for both facilities.   [board chair, successful merger]

One popular department to consolidate is patient accounting. Armed with a comprehensive computer system and knowledgeable staff, a single service department can provide high-volume, well-coordinated patient billing—if the employees who are coming together understand why they have to do so and are given the latitude to forge their own working relationships:

> THE BUSINESS OFFICE, for example, is almost equidistant between the two facilities. We removed the business offices from each campus and put them at one site, with one supervisor.
>
> [employee, successful merger]

> ELEVEN OF US—the billing department—were brought over here from Hospital X. We're all together now, the billing staffs from Hospital X and Hospital Y. I don't think we had any problem combining. We get along pretty well. Basically, after the awkwardness wore off—after a couple weeks—I don't think there was any problem at all.   [employee, eventual failed merger]

> THE CONSOLIDATED PATIENT accounting office is the same system, but it's set up two different ways. What confusion! We do one hospital's billing, stop, and do the other hospital's billing, because there are certain things that are not done the same way. We're both getting paid, but we've got to find a common ground. There is a lot of work to be done yet.
>
> [employee, financially struggling merger]

> WE HAD BEEN in the middle of the city, and there was no place to walk. I loved the hospital, and I liked going there, and it didn't bother me to drive there—but this is just a nicer area to be in. It's brighter and nicer. We love it.
>
> [employee, financially struggling merger]

With any consolidation of hospital departments, management consolidation generally occurs as well. Managers who before a merger had been comfortable in the seeming security of their one department suddenly find themselves overseeing two functional areas at two separate locations after the merger. This change takes its toll not only on the managers themselves but also on the staff members who need access to them:

> SOME MANAGERS HAVE gone over to the other hospital, and some managers from there have come over here. It's been a trade-off.
> [employee, successful merger]

> WE SHARE ADMINISTRATIVE people now. Sometimes the one you want might be at the other hospital, but it's just a different extension on the phone. They're not on the other side of the earth.
> [physician, successful merger]

> BEFORE THE ALLIANCE, we had many more managers, of course. Over the last few years, we've lost many managers. So the managers are now taking care of two and three departments. Before the alliance, we had better communication and much more support from our managers. Now, it's a little frustrating—just a little bit frustrating—because sometimes it takes a lot longer to speak to your manager. Maybe your manager is over at the other hospital or over in another department, and you can sense her frustration.
> [employee, eventual failed merger]

Nurses also face many challenges from postmerger consolidation. The following comment is from an RN who had worked for more than 25 years at one hospital and found herself assigned to a patient unit at the partner hospital after a merger. She was frustrated initially but then came to accept the situation:

> WHEN OUR UNIT moved to the partner site, I felt like a new student again. You know, "I need this." "Well, order it." Everything's different. I felt like I had 32,000 questions. But everybody's been great. As far as that goes, the support system's been excellent. The people who were designated to give the support were 100 percent there and made themselves available 24 hours a day.
> [employee, financially struggling merger]

Finally, another RN expressed well the sentiments and those of her colleagues about the merger's forcing change upon them when their unit was relocated:

> WE ALL WONDERED where we were going to go and what was going to happen to us. You know what was involved: fear of the unknown, worries about acceptance of the others and their acceptance of us, wondering if we could integrate all that we'd learned into their policies and activities. But that transition went quite well; there was really no difficulty. We all knew one another, so that helped, and I knew I would still be in the same facility.
>
> [employee, eventual failed merger]

As with anything, time's passing blurs the shock of change. Perhaps it is human nature that we can get used to anything if we have to put up with it long enough. Although safe and secure daily hospital routines give way to the disruption that merger brings, the initial gamut of emotions one day disappears. In time, newer staff members do not even know anything about two separate organizations, but only know the current reality of the one, now-merged hospital. The pain of consolidation is very real, but it is also very temporary. The transition is eased by philosophical underpinnings and communication about what has happened.

INFRASTRUCTURE CONSOLIDATIONS

Just as department consolidations improve operational efficiencies, infrastructure consolidations improve alignment and save money for the merged hospital. It is a daunting task to line up such things as personnel policies, administrative procedures, wage and benefit structures, and computer systems to forge one infrastructure from two. However, infrastructure consolidation must occur before a merger gets too far along. The infrastructure allows the newly merged entity to function. Hospital staff members can go about their daily work without wondering when they will be paid or how much, whether they will ever get a day off and how to do so, or what their pension reward will be for toiling in this new system when they already had pensions under the old system.

Combining benefits packages between merging hospitals is no small task, and the complexity of that task is noted in the following comments:

> WE HAD TO create, from a human resources viewpoint, an infrastructure that really supported people moving between campuses and transferring. We could not have people working side by side with different benefits programs, different pension plans, and different pay structures. So the very first thing we did—and we spent the first year of the consolidation doing it—was establish a new, flexible benefits plan and establish a new paid-time-off plan.
>
> [executive, successful merger]

> WE INSTITUTED A very nice flex benefits program last year, so we standardized our benefit program. We're rolling out a new pension plan, including a matching tax-sheltered annuity–type thing, so there will be defined benefits and supplements. That's going over well. We're trying to be good employers but also trying to educate our employees that these are tough times for healthcare.
>
> [CEO, successful merger]

> FROM DAY ONE we eliminated all the benefits programs, all the wage and salary programs—an enormous number of policies— and within 12 months we reinstated brand-new ones. So we have a brand-new, state-of-the-art wage and salary program. Next spring we'll roll out the second part, the performance management piece, stressing competencies: inclusive cultural and trade-based competency programs.   [executive, financially struggling merger]

> THE PENSION PROGRAM has been restructured—it had been an atrocious pension program—to one in which employees now have no problem participating.   [executive, successful merger]

Because mergers are often seen as merely means to slash expenses, and thus people's jobs, one positive outcome of a merger is increased job opportunities at two campuses instead of one when benefits packages have been aligned:

> TRANSFERABILITY OF STAFF is another good result of our merger. We now have corporatewide benefits plans and things like that which allow people to switch between campuses without taking a major hit on their benefits and having to start over with probationary periods, pension plans, and all those sorts of things.
>
> [executive, successful merger]

Several employees in merged hospitals expressed positive perceptions about the postmerger infrastructure in relation to their benefits packages:

> WE DID LOSE 6 sick days after the merger. We used to get 12 sick days a year; we lost 6 of those. That's the only thing that has changed. That was part of the flex benefits package that was put together since the merger. They wrapped everything into one; they lumped vacation, sick time, and personal holidays into one.
>
> [employee, successful merger]

> IN MY DEPARTMENT, everybody's pay went up, I've heard, because it was evened out from where everyone was.
>
> [employee, eventual failed merger]

> BENEFITS? I THINK benefits are about the same. I think we lost a couple holidays, but I think the benefits are basically the same.
>
> [employee, eventual failed merger]

One very tired nurse spoke with me at the end of her shift. Not only had it been a trying day for her on the job, but also she was not feeling at all positive about her job because of the tensions surrounding the merger:

I THINK THERE were some life insurance changes, but I didn't even read about them yet, and I don't know what's involved. We all got something a couple weeks ago, but I haven't had a chance to look at it yet.   [employee, eventual failed merger]

Finally, human resources—and many other hospital departments—depends heavily on automated record-keeping systems. Computers are an important aspect of hospital infrastructure:

AT THE END of the fiscal year, the two hospitals are now on the same computer system, which we were not a year ago. With everybody on the same computer system, we're all refining our processes to follow that system. Now we will be combining the accounting function into one corporate accounting function that will handle the operations for the two facilities. We'll do the same for the business office.   [executive, successful merger]

Infrastructure consolidations are necessary after a merger as a means to achieve projected cost savings. The infrastructure affects everyone in the organization in regard to pay, benefits and other human resources aspects, and computer automation. Management's challenge is to complete these consolidations fairly, expeditiously, and with sensitivity.

WORKLOAD AND TEAMWORK

Any consolidation usually has one significant result: one combined entity is now doing the work formerly done by two. This process can evolve very smoothly when plenty of hands remain to handle that expanded workload; it unfolds less smoothly when resources are perceived as being insufficient to accomplish the necessary tasks.

The hardships of consolidation fall on managers as well as other employees. Managers who oversee departments that have not physically combined in one location must now travel between the facilities. The driving time can quickly add up each day, and it takes its toll in lost energy and productivity. Challenged managers feel as if they must split themselves to cover more than one place, to keep straight what is occurring at each location, and to maintain quality service at both facilities. Successful teamwork is thus a challenge that not every merger can accomplish.

One challenge is achieving a "sufficient" level of staffing. Hospital volumes are unpredictable on an hourly basis, because people get sick or injured with no regard to a schedule. An emergency room can be booming one minute and have no patients several hours later. Because people expenses are the largest budget item and the most discretionary—compared with other expenses, such as utilities, interest payments, and insurance—staffing is the main target for expense cuts, and employees feel it keenly:

THE ONE NEGATIVE result of the merger that I think everybody feels is that we have a lot more work and fewer people, because people were let go. The other hospital in the merger did not have a midnight shift, and we did. We didn't work weekends, and they did. A lot of people didn't like that, and now we all have to work weekends.   [employee, eventual failed merger]

WE USED TO have monthly staff meetings where we could solve some problems, and we probably have them only twice a year now. I think those monthly staff meetings were very, very important to nursing. We were able to solve minor problems, which helped as we went on with our nursing care. Due to time constraints, now we're lucky if we get an every-other-year evaluation.
                             [employee, eventual failed merger]

SINCE WE MERGED, there's been a lot more work for us, because we do billing for all the other entities. The merger has added a lot more work on *our* part.   [employee, successful merger]

Low staffing levels are a concern not only to employees but also to managers. They have to set the human resources budgets and daily schedules, duties compounded by the added workload of overseeing operations at two locations:

THE MERGER HAS been very challenging for managers—for the ones who have to drive from hospital to hospital. It's difficult to manage and work out of two offices.

[executive, successful merger]

ONE MANAGER SAID, "I'm managing at two sites, and I feel like I have two children. Like with your own kids, they're different, but you love them equally. But it's hard sometimes for employees to get that sense."

[executive, successful merger]

WITH EVERYTHING THAT'S happening, I think the reason we haven't been evaluated is because management hasn't had the time. But if I really mess up, I hear about it.

[employee, eventual failed merger]

Becoming a cohesive team is an elusive goal for the staff communities who must come together from two formerly separate hospitals. A team can be created through positive, "can-do" attitudes and a focus on accomplishing the mission of the functioning departments:

I WILL SAY that since the merger, it's been more positive. Many more departments are working together as a unit, trying to make things better, so we've definitely improved in that regard.

[employee, successful merger]

IS IT HARD to work as one billing office? I wouldn't say it's difficult. It's just throwing a lot of things together—people, personalities, women! You'd understand if you'd worked in a billing office. We get along. I think we've done well. When we were ending our own way of doing what we did all those years, we sat back and looked at it. Then we realized that the other hospital did their job; they got their bills paid. We've done our job our way, and we've gotten our bills paid. We just have to become a team. I don't think there's any big animosity.   [employee, financially struggling merger]

New equipment can be invaluable in keeping a department focused on its mission and in creating higher levels of commitment by staff:

THE PCS ARE brand new for everybody since the merger, and they've made my life grand. I touch a couple keys, and I can put in things I use everyday. I don't have to worry about typing the same thing in every single time. This happened since we moved to this joint location.   [employee, financially struggling merger]

Consolidation of the nursing staff can lead to particularly thorny problems. Nursing is integral in public perceptions of what a hospital is and what it represents. The last seven letters in the word *represents,* however, spell the word *resents,* and all too often after a merger there is resentment from the nursing staff and about the nursing staff. Nursing needs people on its staff to accomplish its essential work:

THE HOSPITAL RUNS a very efficient, lean staff, and sometimes the staff morale and employee morale is a little too tight. We don't have quite enough nurses to do this or that, and that situation has been pretty much a trademark of how the hospital has been operating.   [physician, successful merger]

NURSING HAS BEEN cut; aides have been cut. There are two nurses and one aide for 12 people, and somebody's got to eat sometime. That's my main concern.   [employee, successful merger]

The single best commentary on the daily realities of life in any hospital, merged or not, came from an executive whose level of resentment toward forces beyond his control made him appear ready to give up due to the headaches of matching staffing to daily patient volumes:

> WE'VE GONE THROUGH periods of ups and downs. One minute we're laying off, and the next minute we're hiring. That has not changed.   [executive, eventual failed merger]

Hospitals are experts in teamwork. The critical interconnectedness among departments has always been a hallmark of the caring hospital. Staff members operate under the rule that patients come first—after all, that is why employees are at work.

Hospital mergers do not change that ethic. However, mergers do change the staff outlook toward that ethic: "You mean I have to work alongside that person from that hospital? Right here on my floor? Those people never took care of patients like we do." This is a familiar scenario, and it is only accentuated by the burdens of the additional workload that often accompanies a merger.

Such a situation requires great sensitivity on the part of the organization's leaders. Board members do not necessarily spend much time inside the walls of the hospital they are governing. Executives are in the hospital, yet their responsibilities span a multitude of areas, with only one of them being staff morale. Department managers thus often feel they lack a support structure that would bolster their daily decision making.

PERCEPTIONS OF CARE

It is crucial that the perception of hospital care, both before and after a merger, be positive or even improved from previous positive perceptions. The voices about this topic are almost unanimous in stating that after a merger, care remains high in quality and either as good as or better than it was before the merger. It is comforting that despite all the changes on the business side, hospitals give the steady, respected, and traditional good care that has been their hallmark over the years.

One executive begins the dialog by describing the schizophrenic reality that is daily hospital management:

> I THINK THAT it can be summed up by, "Patients come first." I think that's the way it has always been. We want patients to have the best care that they can get, but at the same time it is a business also.   [executive, successful merger]

How do the patients themselves perceive their care? Does post-merger care stack up to the memory of care before a merger? The following patient, who refers to a successful merger, was not interested as much in why the merger had occurred as in the present situation:

> PEOPLE WHO DON'T go to the doctor—they could care less about the merger. Once they start going to the doctor, they're going to find a much better system since the merger. Now patients can jump from one hospital to another without a whole lot of hassle if they need to. And the hospitals give you the best care they can. I hope that's why they merged in the first place.
>   [patient, successful merger]

Another patient—this one at a hospital whose merger eventually failed—wasn't so positive:

> THE STAFF'S ATTITUDE was really good, but I guess they don't have enough time. Maybe the hospital is short of help. It takes a while to get personal things handled. For example, I was here a whole day before I got a towel or washcloth, and I asked three different times. It seemed unorganized.
>   [patient, eventual failed merger]

Positive comments came from patients in two mergers with very different outcomes. The good points prevailed nevertheless:

I LIVE NEARBY, and this hospital is my first preference. It's close to home, I don't have to pay for parking—it's got its advantages. And I think it has a good, rounded staff. Without that, a hospital doesn't stay around too long, believe me.

[patient, financially struggling merger]

I COULDN'T BE more impressed with the caregivers. Everyone is very nice, very knowledgeable, exemplary. They are really a great group. I see a big difference from my past experiences. Everyone is courteous, prompt, and can't do enough for you. I like that.

[patient, successful merger]

The final comment is from a husband and wife; the wife was a patient, and the husband was visiting. They were very articulate healthcare consumers who had spent much time and effort reviewing their choices for health insurance and felt personally unaffected by the merger:

WE DON'T SEE any difference. Nothing has changed. But we haven't participated enough to know all the various services and whether something has changed or not.　　[patient, successful merger]

A hospital is not a large, sprawling building, the latest MRI scanner, or even a nicely decorated lobby. Because perception is reality, a hospital is each person who comes in contact with a patient/customer, and the sentiment toward that hospital flows directly out through feelings toward caregivers, housekeeping aides, dietary food servers, and even repairers who enter a patient's room. Hospital mergers cause great disruptions in organizational structure, but keeping those disruptions invisible to patients allows the mission to be achieved.

FALLOUT

Less of a Family Feeling, More Impersonal

Society expects newly merged hospitals to keep going and not miss a beat, to keep any consternation hidden, and to serve the community as always. A glimpse inside merged organizations reveals that in reality, change takes time to be accepted, to be overcome, and to be conquered with daily operations that surpass the old.

Hospitals traditionally see themselves as a family. With the doors open 365 days year, 24 hours a day, the hospital staff musters relationships that create bonds for life, as each person, every day, contributes skills that literally mean life and death. The sense of teamwork and supporting coworkers is very strong. Recreating that sense of family and personal relationships is difficult in a merger when each staff member's life is disrupted by the need to adjust immediately to new coworkers. One physician with a negative observation about the present situation still holds an optimistic view for the future:

> THE WORST THING is that some of the positive aspects of the hospital, I think, have been lost in combining with the partner hospital. I think it's become more impersonal. But I think some of that might be just the transition, so maybe in the long run it will be better.   [physician, successful merger]

It is natural for employees to long for the way things had been before the merger. We are human beings, not robots programmed to respond according to a certain formula. This business office worker laments several losses:

> I MISS THE closeness of the people. I walk around the hospital now, and I don't know half the people I run into. They're from different places. I hear of someone in upper management and

wonder, "Who is that person?" I don't think we're well informed about new people—that type of thing—and I don't like that part. But I guess the thing that causes me the most dissatisfaction is that we aren't a close-knit group anymore.

[employee, successful merger]

Because of the many new priorities for leaders after a merger, one area easy to neglect is sensitivity to employees who are still going on in their daily roles. The touches of kindness and appreciation that may have existed before a merger are often forgotten in the crush of rapid change. This employee was very sad after a merger to think that all her work was in vain, since no one seemed to care:

THERE WAS MORE caring in the past about people's work. Sometimes somebody would come up and say, "Hey, you're doing a good job." Sometimes people need that, you know. But now it feels like we're doing the work, but nobody's even noticing.

[employee, financially struggling merger]

Whoever could capture the essence of the premerger hospitals, bottle it up, and create a magic potion for postmerger entities would become a billionaire immediately. This housekeeping worker was near tears relating the differences between "her" hospital and the merged organization:

ABOUT THE MERGER, I am definitely disappointed. Even though I knew it was inevitable, I feel there was a unique quality about the old hospital that is not lost but that's been sort of reassigned. It's sad. It was gradual.   [employee, financially struggling merger]

Although working in an organization that considered itself successful after its merger, this RN was not happy with the state of affairs:

I DON'T THINK communication is any better since the merger. I don't think anything's a whole lot different. It's a lot less like family, which it used to be. We knew one another. I guess I don't feel it's as warm as it used to be when it was just our hospital.

[employee, successful merger]

Friendliness is not familyness, as this medical records clerk stated:

EVERYBODY SAYS "HELLO"—people I don't know. I walk down the hall, and everybody says good morning. I think they're friendly, but I don't think it's family.   [employee, eventual failed merger]

Two RNs expressed great sadness and personal frustration at working inside their hospitals after the merger. After many years in familiar units and among familiar coworkers both had to move to another location. The pain in their voices does not translate well on paper:

PERSONALLY, I DON'T feel good. Some days I'd leave. And I absolutely love nursing. I always have—even at its worst, when we had an oncology patient, I could make the patient who was dying feel some self-worth. I just love nursing. But I just don't feel that here. Somewhere it's gotten lost. I don't feel really good about my job now. I realize we've had a change and things are different, but I don't feel that accountability is there. I'm having a really hard time with that, because I feel I should be accountable.

[employee, financially struggling merger]

I PROBABLY FELT more "in the know" at Hospital X, only because I had been there for so long. I knew everything; I knew everybody; I knew where everything was. Here I don't know where anything is. I don't know where the nurse is; I don't know where the lab is; I don't know where x-ray is. I don't know the place, so I can't feel right at

home, because I don't know where I am right now! I don't know if
I know how to get back to my department!

[employee, eventual failed merger]

Postmerger fallout that is due to impersonalization and a less
familylike atmosphere is very real to those who spend, at times,
more than half their available 24-hour days on hospital duty. Ownership develops over the years as employees forge bonds and
friendships with coworkers and the hospital itself, and their commitment to their jobs is extremely high. Loss of that ownership as
a result of a merger is difficult, if not almost impossible, to re-
store, but successful hospital mergers somehow get close.

Difficulty Achieving Acceptance

One of the greatest challenges in a merger is achieving throughout the organization the same degree of acceptance and faith in
the merger as is felt by the leaders who made the decision to merge.
Those leaders had months—and perhaps years—to realize that a
merger was necessary. They have had the luxury of time to study
the concept of merger and then to decide it is the best thing for
the community and the hospitals themselves. Others in the organization who hear of the merger decision through an announcement of some type, no matter how carefully crafted the announcement is, cannot appreciate the analysis and soul searching that
went into that message. The news hits—and everyone feels hit.

Once the announcement of merger has been made, the leaders
are ready to implement consolidation plans and launch all the
initiatives they have dreamed about during the entire premerger
stage. It is no wonder that everyone else has a difficult time catching that enthusiasm.

Acceptance of a merger by physicians is critically important.
Physicians were a critical element in this merger that did not stay
together:

I THINK MERGING hospitals must have physician buy-in; there's a critical mass of physicians that is needed, or else the merger won't get community buy-in. I'm not sure what that number is yet, but it's something at or slightly over 50 percent. The majority of physicians must be willing to say, "We think this makes sense for our community." Without that, the merger is not going to get community support, because the physicians will sabotage all of the efforts—all of the communication efforts; all of the advertising, marketing, and promotional efforts—all the way through the system, all the way through the process.   [CEO, eventual failed merger]

I SEE OUR physicians as the most difficult group—the greatest obstacle right now. The employees, I think, will come around when they see what can be affected by it, but the strongest group that can really pull us down right now is the physicians.

[trustee, eventual failed merger]

Acceptance of the merger by employees takes time—possibly more time than might be expected or even available. Acceptance is derived from trust, and trust flows from predictability and security. Mergers, however, provide anything but that in the early days:

A LOT OF the employees talked about the grieving process that has to take place. A lot of that did take place, and in some people is still taking place. They have trouble accepting and thinking of themselves as being part of a system. If you ask them where they work, they would say Hospital X or Hospital Y. I don't think they think in terms of the new system.

[executive, successful merger]

I THINK THE jury is out for many employees here, and one of the reasons is that we're still finalizing benefits across the board. Until the benefits get uniform, the employees will be looking at pros and cons of what we used to have and what we have now.

[employee, successful merger]

One human resources executive described why acceptance of a merger was low:

> UNFORTUNATELY, THE HOSPITAL organization, from day one, for no good reason, in my opinion, adopted the posture of being the victim. It caused some people to quit. Now, none of those things have come to pass, and it's been well over a year. Most people are still working. People haven't been harmed en masse or anything like that. [executive, financially struggling merger]

These comments lead to the obvious questions: Why did that perception arise? What was done to precipitate it? What was being done to dispel it?

It is difficult to share and spread a hospital's vision in times of peace, when employees have nothing unusual or particularly stressful to consume their interests. Sharing the vision in times of war, such as after a merger, becomes a monumental task. This executive expressed that well:

> I WOULD SAY the largest disappointment or frustration I have is our failure to bring the people of the organizations along with us on the journey as quickly as we would have liked to. They are not totally in step with this merger, and that kind of retards everything we're trying to accomplish in the organization.
> [executive, financially struggling merger]

Finally, an RN who struggled to understand the reasons for her organization's merger and to accept it got to the point where she stopped trying to analyze it herself and let those in charge handle the situation:

> I'M NOT A business woman, OK? So when those business changes are being made, I'm really trusting that those people are really the experts in making business decisions.
> [employee, successful merger]

Acceptance of a merger takes time. Merger leaders know this and are not intimidated by the daunting task it represents. That does not mean those leaders have an easy road to travel—just a worthwhile one.

Lack of Planning

Planning is one of the most critical duties of management, but it is a responsibility that is not carried out as well as it could be. There just are not enough crystal balls to go around, and the ones that are available do not give a clear view into the future. Thinking into the future is very hard work. It takes tremendous effort to stretch one's thoughts into the sky, place oneself there, and determine all the consequences of the decision about to be made. Questions must be answered: Who will be affected, and how? Why should this decision be made? How do I know this is the correct decision, given all the alternatives?

That analysis does seem like a lot of effort, but ignoring it before a merger decision results in a good deal more effort. Backing up from an ill-planned merger or amending a well-intentioned merger idea that simply did not get the necessary srutiny has far-reaching consequences. The merger voices on this topic are worth hearing, as the painful experiences they share come from having been at a decision point and not projecting forward well enough.

One trustee had a very candid view of the lack of planning in his merger situation. You will note his voice change at the end—from the third person (blaming *them*) to the first person *we* (accepting responsibility):

> THEY MADE A decision almost overnight. They brought all the boards together and told them what they had to do in order to have a vote. That was absurd. You just don't do that. And they found out—we found out—the hard way.
>
> [trustee, eventual failed merger]

One community representative was critical about the manner in which the merger leaders in her community approached the project. She was reeling from things that she had heard locally. Although she personally supported the hospital merger as the best thing for the community, she felt that some of the personal disputes could have been avoided had there been more forthrightness in the planning and communication process:

THE BIGGEST CRITICISM, or the most negative thing, was not having a well-thought-out plan, not thinking it through as much as we might have in order to really make the merger work. To build trust, an organization has to make its promises clear and stick to those promises.   [community representative, successful merger]

This board chair had invested so much of his personal reputation in making the merger come to pass that it was particularly sad to hear him talk about how long-range plans could not be implemented because of the extreme financial problems that arose:

I HAD ALWAYS envisioned that after this affiliation agreement took place it would take a couple years before a clinical consolidation plan would really be implemented. Well, that was moved up considerably due to finances, and it was soon announced what this plan would be. That's when all hell broke loose. That would have been expected two years from then anyway, but at least we would have given the employees and the people in the community the opportunity to understand what the health system was, what it was trying to accomplish. As it was, we were just out there trying to play defense, and we never got to play offense. That's why we got in the mess we were in this winter.

[board chair, eventual failed merger]

A nurse in the same merger had an opposite frustration: she was tired of the indecision and wanted no more time to elapse before the clinical consolidations were accomplished. Announcements had been made one way, retracted, reissued about a different decision, and then not acted on. She felt that the merger planning was very poorly done, and she spoke the sentiments of many employees in the organization who just wanted to "know their fate," as she expressed it:

> I JUST WISH the decision makers would make up their minds. I wish they would just do it. They say they're going to do this, this, and that. And they say they're doing it for the good of the community, and for the good of the hospital. I know they are under a lot of pressure, but I just wish they'd do it.
>
> [employee, eventual failed merger]

For employees, hearing about a merger and its reasons is one thing; life goes on. It is quite another thing when a particular change affects an individual staff member. Employees who are affected by postmerger changes on a day-to-day basis respond strongly to a lack of premerger planning: If I'm working in a new or strange environment, am I prepared to do so? And who has taken the time to make sure that I am prepared? This RN expressed it well:

> I THINK ONE of my biggest problems with the merger was that I did not feel the nurses from the other hospital were adequately prepared to come and work in this system. They were expected to come over here and be functional, using our charts, our policies, and our procedures. We give different medications. I was an advocate for getting them more orientation. I was never really given an explanation as to why they were not better prepared, but some of them came over for a day or two and shadowed. But we function very, very differently. We keep the charts right outside the patients' rooms. We do our own medications and primary nursing. We're

not used to residents—that's another issue. I think they felt lost for the first few weeks. And of course that caused a lot of anxiety on their part. It was frustrating for me to know that they were not adequately prepared. And the rest of the staff sees that; they know that.   [employee, financially struggling merger]

Finally, planning is multifaceted and obviously includes decisions regarding top staff. Although his was a successful merger, this CEO had one regret when it came to establishing the postmerger top management team and going forward:

I THINK I would have faced some of the senior management issues early on. I think it was a painful year because we hadn't. And while we did OK, we didn't do as well in the first year as we could have. We made up a lot of ground in the second year. I have a file that's called "Noah's Ark" because we had two of each executive still working and on the job. I think if I had anything to think through and do over again, it would be to streamline top management.

It is always easy to look back and say what should have been done differently. Merger leadership does not come with a built-in crystal ball. However, time and effort devoted to planning pay untold dividends as a merger unfolds and takes on an identity of its own.

Uncertainty and Staff Outmigration

Hospitals are under tremendous pressures on a daily basis. They face myriad challenges to operations: reimbursement cutbacks, changing delivery modes from inpatient to outpatient care, finding ways to decrease expenses to match the change in patient volume and reimbursement, growing public perception of a hospital as a business and not a care institution first and foremost, increased regulatory interference, and on and on. Those pressures are some of the very same catalysts that cause hospital mergers in the first place.

Persons who work in hospitals and stay there have learned to cope with that uncertainty. However, once a new element of change is introduced in the form of a merger, the equation changes dramatically. Thoughts immediately turn inward: How will this merger affect me? As would be expected, some employees answer this question with their feet, and others respond with more questions.

After a merger, a key question on employees' minds is job security. Note the differences in the following comments from employees in both failed and successful mergers:

> I WORRY ABOUT whether or not I'm going to keep a job. I would assume that if the hospitals combine forces completely when the merger is done, they're not going to need a lot of us.
>
> [employee, eventual failed merger]

> I THINK MY only concern was that I would not lose my job—that the organization would not downsize. And they assured us many, many, many, many, many times that they would not do that. The only way downsizing would happen would be through attrition, and they've stuck with that. They've been very encouraging and very informative, and I never really felt too threatened.
>
> [employee, successful merger]

The prospect of living with more change on a daily basis creates added apprehensions. Two RNs from different organizations expressed uncertainty caused by change in general:

> I DON'T THINK people's support for the merger would have anything to do with the affiliation—the employees don't mind that. I

think the problem is that people don't want to change the way they were doing things. That's human nature.

[employee, financially struggling merger]

I THINK SOME of us older ones are worse than the younger ones; we don't like to see change. And we have a tendency to think that every time there's a change, it's negative. And people tend to respond in an uproar before they really get all the facts. They rely on rumors and things like that. [employee, successful merger]

In a merger, apprehensions surround not only the decision to merge itself but also the merger partner. In many cases, two seemingly bitter enemies find themselves on the same side of the service table, and this is not an easy situation:

THE EMPLOYEES FELT apprehension about the merger. Maybe some felt relief that there was going to be a partnership. There was a lot of uncertainty about where things were going to fall. In many cases there was judgment and some criticism: "Why does Hospital X get med/surg? They're very different from us. We are an inner-city hospital, and they are in the rolling hills of the suburbs." Those were just perceptions, but as we know, perceptions can be awfully real to people. [executive, financially struggling merger]

I THINK ONE of the biggest fears that everyone has is that we are going to be sucked up by the partner hospital because it is supposedly bigger than us. Also, people fear that because the other hospital had financial problems, we are going to get drawn into some of their bad decisions or whatever and, as a result, end up in the red. [employee, successful merger]

Mergers often bring management changes. These changes can be forced or voluntary, but in either case they have sweeping effects. The following comments are typical of how change in management was received in a merger that was not coming together as well as had been expected:

> CHANGE IS ALWAYS hard. I was very happy working with the manager I was working with. I had a lot of personal anxiety about working with the new one, but things are working out fine.
>
> [employee, financially struggling merger]

> THE MANAGEMENT STAFF here at Hospital X is almost all gone, so it's obvious how they viewed the merger. The rest of the staff were more concerned about losing their jobs—not having work— than blending or going with each other.
>
> [board chair, financially struggling merger]

One comment from an employee sums up the prevalent feeling of many in the field today regarding the pace of changes. The interviewee was a dedicated housekeeping worker who wanted nothing more than to do a good job each day. She had a very positive attitude toward the merger of her hospital:

> WHAT IF THEY start closing things? You know, who's to say that it won't happen? In the health field, you never know. It changes every day. You don't even want to take a day off, because you don't know what tomorrow will bring!   [employee, successful merger]

The outmigration of staff is a by-product of uncertainty, as well as certainty. Uncertainty breeds insecurity and pushes staff to look for jobs elsewhere. Certainty projects an image of what the merged organization looks like, and staff members quickly decide whether or not to remain and share the vision.

Both successful and less-than-successful mergers had positive aspects (for example, perceptions of good-quality care and successful department consolidations) as well as negative aspects (for example, less of a family feeling, difficulty achieving acceptance, problems due to lack of planning, and uncertainty and staff outmigration). Successful mergers face the same challenges as failed mergers, but the successful ones are able to navigate more decisively.

What We Have Heard

Condition	Successful Merger	Less-Than-Successful Merger
Communication		
• Open	yes	no
• Adequate	yes	no
• More than before merger	yes	no
• Frequent	yes	no
Medical staff link		
• Cross-credentialing	yes	yes
• Joint activities	yes	no
• Physicians supportive	yes	no
• Physician concern about clinical consolidation	no	yes
Department consolidations	yes	yes
Infrastructure consolidations	yes	yes
Workload and teamwork	yes	yes
Positive perceptions of care	yes	yes
Fallout		
• Less of a family feeling, more impersonal	yes	yes

(continued on following page)

What We Have Heard
(*continued*)

Condition	Successful Merger	Less-Than-Successful Merger
• Difficulty achieving acceptance	yes	yes
• Lack of planning	yes	yes
• Uncertainty and staff outmigration	yes	yes

Clues and Hallmarks

Did you notice any particular characteristics that gave the successful mergers an edge? Why would the postmerger conditions be similar in the successful mergers and the failed mergers?

Chapter 7

DECIDING HOW TO
HANDLE EMPLOYEES

AVOID STAFF REDUCTIONS

A merger affords the opportunity to achieve efficiencies in operations. Salaries and wages, the single largest expense in any hospital's budget, is the prime target for savings. Any merger involves service and departmental consolidations, and the question of how to handle any excess number of employees needs to be approached delicately and its many facets appreciated.

The fears brought about by the merger itself manifest themselves concretely when staff reductions occur, thus spreading the areas of "fallout" described in the previous chapter throughout the organization. Some organizations choose to reduce staffing expense through attrition, but the trade-off of that policy is a delayed realization of operational cost savings for a merger.

One successful merger organization sent a strong message throughout the newly merged hospital that its past no-layoff policy would continue. This message was seen, believed, and supported:

THERE'S STILL A no-layoff policy for employees. The organization has always said no layoffs, no layoffs—and there have been no layoffs. And I think the hospital administration has kept its word. In the 19 years I've been here, there have been no layoffs.

[employee, successful merger]

Not all employees feel so secure. The hospital may not have a clearcut position on layoffs. In these cases, other planning issues are raised besides job security:

I THINK THE initial response of many employees was the question of layoffs. That was their first major concern. They wondered what services would still be here, and what services would be at the other campus. The employees worried what the implications would be for them.   [physician, financially struggling merger]

Attrition works in many cases. It is an approach that makes sense to persons within the organization, and it is a generally well-supported policy. These comments are from successful mergers:

WE REALLY HAVEN'T had any layoffs or what we call cutbacks. It's been done through attrition. As people leave, we haven't replaced them, so we kind of come up with new ways to do our services.

[employee, successful merger]

THERE ARE NO layoffs, no firings or anything—but attrition can really work. Employees are told they'll always have a job. They are told that they may have to work at different places, but they'll always have a job. This allows management to give security to employees.   [physician, successful merger]

THERE WERE SOME job losses due to the merger, but the majority have occurred at the management level. As individuals leave, we choose not to replace them. We didn't boot out anybody that I can think of off the top of my head specifically because of the merger.

We have labor unions we have to deal with, so it's not as simple as that.   [executive, successful merger]

A policy akin to attrition is brokering employees to other jobs within the merger system. When this method is possible, it goes far in establishing the merged hospital as credible and viable:

THE LAYOFFS HERE, I believe, have been minimal. I think that every attempt has been made to re-deploy employees whose positions have been eliminated. I know that when we closed a unit that wasn't doing well, the employees received a list of all the open positions in the system. We said, "Here's what we have available. Feel free to bid if you're qualified. We certainly will give you preferential consideration." The system has really done a good job with that method.   [executive, successful merger]

Most organizations hope that layoffs will never have to occur, but in reality, they often must. The disbelief and mistrust in the voices of the following three employees is lost in print:

I NEVER THOUGHT the third floor would close. I had been there for 19 of my years here at the hospital. I never thought it could happen, because there had been talk in the past about hospitals closing and layoffs, and nothing ever happened. But this time it came true.   [employee, eventual failed merger]

WE HAD A lot of bad apples that left. The people who were always complaining left. They complained and complained and complained. They left. The hospital got rid of them, or whatever.
                    [employee, financially struggling merger]

THERE'S A GREAT antagonism at the hospital, I think, between the employees and administration. The employees didn't trust the administration, and I think that's why it was such a hyped-up atmosphere. Obviously, there were a lot of layoffs, and people were never really told why.   [employee, eventual failed merger]

The board chair of a merger that is still struggling was torn between feeling good about the positive things the merger had already accomplished and feeling terrible knowing what was yet to come—all in the name of financial success:

IF YOU ASKED me a couple of weeks ago, I would have thought attaining merger goals was good. If you had asked me since last week, I would have been a little leery because of the new staff cuts that are coming.   [board chair, financially struggling merger]

INCREASE JOB OPPORTUNITIES

One of the indisputably positive by-products of a hospital merger is the partnership of the formerly separate campuses that creates doubled job avenues as long as the consolidated services volume warrants the staff. Furthermore, overhead departments, such as maintenance and housekeeping, are still needed to function at both locations, even if a staff reduction occurs.

Two nurses echoed very positive comments about the broadened job opportunities afforded by a merger:

JOBS HAVE BEEN listed for different positions, more positions now than there used to be. There's been more opportunity for people to get different jobs.   [employee, successful merger]

DUE TO THE fact that postings are campuswide for both campuses, we know what's going on or what's available throughout the organization. Communications accelerate that way. Before, there were two separate campuses and no communications.

[employee, successful merger]

A housekeeping employee who felt enormous loyalty to her hospital was philosophical about what the merger could do for her coworkers (but not herself, because she planned to do no moving):

> THIS HOSPITAL WOULD still be my home base. But it's nice to know that there are two campuses, so we have even more opportunities. [employee, successful merger]

This RN spoke freely about her support of the merger. She realized that it made sense in the community, and she supported it in talking to less-trusting colleagues:

> I THINK THAT six months ago, everybody was scared to death that they wouldn't have a job. Since we've been taken over, we have felt a little more secure in the fact that we can be flexible and go to either hospital. Seniority was carried over, which had been another major concern. [employee, eventual failed merger]

Finally, one long-tenured nurse shared her mixed emotions about a profession she dearly loved and a hospital that had been home to her for 25 years:

> DO I SUPPORT the merger? Well, that depends. Do you want the practical side? Do you want the emotional side? Do you want the professional side? From the emotional side, we'd run right back home to Hospital X. Professionally, I'd like to continue to grow. Practically, we will be able to provide better care.
> [employee, financially struggling merger]

The people affected by a merger see it more positively when they realize that more, rather than fewer, jobs will be available. Some people in an organization come to that realization more readily and easily than others.

GIVE MORE AUTONOMY

Empowerment has been one of the most important concepts in management literature and thought for the past decade. It connotes principles of management that are worth attaining in any organization: a sense of security for employees who feel comfortable enough to take charge of a situation, a sense of trust on the part of management that employees will make good decisions on behalf of the company, and increased satisfaction on the part of customers whose needs are handled at the immediate level. Some organizations have adopted the phrase "You see it, you own it, you take care of it."

Hospitals have traditionally been empowered organizations to a point. The clinical personnel, especially nurses and technicians, have always been expected to follow their best judgment regarding patient care (for example, deciding to telephone a physician to report a change in patient condition). The hospital world, however, is governed by elaborate policies, procedures, and protocols to guide the daily work of employees. These rules are necessary to ensure the highest possible quality of care in all instances and all matter of service departments. Hospitals have never been "incubator" businesses, as are computer technology companies, for example, where new ideas and constant creative thinking are the norm.

True empowerment in a hospital manifests itself in autonomy: the ability of employees to work both independently and collaboratively with other departments as needed. Mergers afford the ready-made opportunity for hospitals to give more autonomy to employees, as the following voices relate. However, this increased autonomy occurs, perhaps, more by default and as a by-product of the merger itself. Employees have to think more for themselves because management is busy with many other things.

The expression of freedom to do one's job is evident in the following comments from employees. Their tone of voice is one of enthusiasm—not skepticism or criticism—and they have renewed interest in jobs that are more meaningful and fulfilling:

> I DID ENJOY my job before the merger, but I felt like I was crowded into a really small area of the job. Now I just pretty much can do my job and develop new things.   [employee, successful merger]

> I NOW REPORT to somebody else who is miles away down the road and who is not here everyday. But she still gives me the freedom and flexibility to do whatever I have to do to get the job done.
> [employee, successful merger]

> WE DON'T HAVE anybody looking over our shoulders all the time, and that's good. It's really a good place to work. And that hasn't changed since the merger.
> [employee, successful merger]

I remember one business office clerk's excitement over a new accounts receivable progress graph her department had begun using just three months before. The charted trend was fewer days in accounts receivable, and the staff had been rewarded with a pizza party:

> UNDER OUR OLD supervisor there was limited independence; under the new supervisor there's a lot of independence. I get a lot more accomplished. We keep track of our accounts receivable on a chart, and we're proud that it's going down.
> [employee, successful merger]

This housekeeping worker would embody the definition of empowerment if it could ever take the shape of a human being:

> NOW I THINK things are more open. If our supervisor is at the partner or another facility, we are allowed to take on the responsibility of calling somebody to fill in where jobs are not being completed, or we just do it ourselves.   [employee, successful merger]

Despite the eventual failure of the merger involved, another housekeeping worker was grateful for the positive changes in daily routines that came from being given more responsibility because of the less-frequent presence of her manager:

> TO TELL YOU the truth, in the last four or five years, I guess we've become more independent because we don't have the backup. We just can't run to our managers for every little thing, because they're not available. So we make more decisions ourselves.
>   [employee, eventual failed merger]

Another housekeeping worker had relocated from a hospital in a very large city. She felt that that hospital was impersonal and unfriendly, as well as having lower standards. She was delighted with her move and was totally supportive of the style of management after the merger:

> THE BOSSES ARE not constantly on my back or anything. And if I'm doing something wrong, they will tell me—they just pull me aside. They don't embarrass me or anything. I think that's wonderful. That's great.   [employee, financially struggling merger]

If empowerment of employees is a desired state in order to fulfill customer service expectations, the autonomy afforded through a hospital merger can be one means to provide that. Whether because of staffing cuts as departments are consolidated or less direct involvement by managers who are stretched to cover more than one venue, employees can think for themselves frequently after the merger.

Employee issues of staffing levels, layoffs, increased job opportunities, and autonomy are crucial in a merger. With the exception of avoiding staff reductions, those employee issues are similarly handled in the new organizational structure of both successful and less-than-successful mergers. Opportunities for employees usually increase in a merged hospital organization that has multiple service sites, whether or not the outcome is successful.

What We Have Heard

Goal	Successful Merger	Less-Than-Successful Merger
Avoid staff reductions	yes	no
Increase job opportunities	yes	yes
Give more autonomy	yes	yes

Clues and Hallmarks

Is avoiding staff reductions possible only when mergers show positive financial performance? Did you detect anything in the successful merger comments that indicates better ways of handling employee issues? What are the negative consequences of employees having more freedom to do their work?

Chapter 8

CREATING A NEW IDENTITY

A name is critically important to an organization. From a name, identity is derived and reputation is created. The act of naming launches an entity along its path in history, as generations to come will use whatever name is given.

Hospitals that merge bring their own names with their own histories. Many hospitals have long histories, with foundings in the late 1800s or early 1900s, and thus their names have been part of the common community language for years. The merger, depending on how it is structured, may create the need for the joining partners to take on new names that reflect the new relationship.

Philosophically, leaders grapple with the dilemma of whether to downplay the merger and continue to emphasize the existing hospital names or highlight the merger and use new names for the hospitals. A merger also has the inherent challenge of developing its new identity in the minds of those who are part of the new organization. The following merger voices address these aspects of merger.

One method expressed by people from several merged entities was to come out charging with the new name, to use the name of the merger from that point forward, and to focus on the merger as the key to the future:

THE MERGER NAME is out there now. I daresay that a year ago, people would have asked, "What's that?"

[executive, successful merger]

WE'RE NOT DOING individual hospital ads any longer. Everything is run as the merger name, so all of our marketing efforts are toward the merger organization now. I think that's made a big difference in terms of the community's recognizing us as one instead of recognizing us as individual units.

[executive, successful merger]

DO AWAY WITH the names of both hospitals, and just call them by the merger name—have everything coming out of the health system. Get rid of the building names so people can get that out of their minds, and just worry about the quality—the services we're providing. Don't get attached to those buildings because of history. And do this while it's quiet. Don't wait until we make decisions, because then people are going to choose sides.

[trustee, eventual failed merger]

A differing opinion, though, is that the name of the merger has no value for daily operations. Retaining use of the individual hospital names preserves the identity and history of two long-standing institutions in a community. One hospital executive pointed out that people in outlying towns did not even recognize the name of the merger organization:

THE NAME RECOGNITION is still Hospital X and Hospital Y, which is fine with us, because those are the names. They are pillars in the community, and ones that we never want to lose. The name of the merger entity is a management group.

[executive, successful merger]

One of the most difficult tasks in a merger, though, no matter what names are used for the merged hospital, is to create the feeling and sense that the new organization is truly merged and unified. This struggle takes longer than anyone would ever expect. Turning separate, individual identities and cultures forged over decades into one jointly held identity takes years:

I JUST THINK that our organization needs to create a *we* approach instead of a *they* approach. Sometimes when I say *we*, people aren't sure what I'm talking about, because they haven't identified with *we* yet. [executive, eventual failed merger]

MOST EMPLOYEES AT the hospital and the medical staff still think of *them* and *they*, and they still want to point fingers. Now it's slowly going away, but there is still some of that—even, quite frankly, at the board level. Some board members still think of themselves as protecting one hospital or the other.

[executive, successful merger]

EVEN THE USE of pronouns reflects people's feelings. We've tried to work with people on not saying, "*We* at Hospital X and *they* at Hospital Y" and vice versa. We try to get people to think about it more in terms of *us*. But it's challenging. On any given day, there continue to be those kinds of feelings and issues. And there are still barriers. There are a lot of information systems barriers and payroll systems and financial systems in which we still have two di=erent ways of doing things. [executive, successful merger]

Perhaps one of the most tangible examples of the effort to break down the barriers is the following comment from an employee who wanted to support the merger completely but saw little relief from "stupid" things that the organization did:

I REMEMBER LAST Christmas, during the holidays, we had a holiday dinner. One campus served turkey, and the other campus served beef—and there was a great big craziness about what kind of meat was served. To me, that's ridiculous, but for our employees it was symbolic. [employee, financially struggling merger]

Creating a new identity is the main task of a newly merged organization. Doing so presupposes that everyone understands and accepts why the merger was effected in the first place, and it represents the bridge between the past (separate hospitals) and the future (one smoothly functioning, mission-oriented, joined hospital). Whichever method of creating that identity is selected, the overriding principle of the organization must be to do what will bring it the most long-term benefits—even if the immediate path is painful.

Clues and Hallmarks

What is the process used to create an identity for a merged entity? Is it better to select a totally new name for the merged entity, or can a combination of the existing names work as well?

What is the value of emotions attached to the premerger names? Can this be harnessed in the new entity?

Chapter 9

UNDERSTANDING WHAT HAS BEEN CREATED

A MECCA OF CARE AND QUALITY

The true synergy in a hospital merger manifests itself in the intrinsic mission of hospitals: providing medical care at an optimal level of quality. Despite the myriad reasons to effect a merger in the first place, the ability to raise that mission to a higher plane by virtue of the merger itself is a significant and worthwhile accomplishment for the community served. The merger voices accentuate this positive aspect of merger.

Board members have the overall responsibility for overseeing the quality of care provided in their hospitals, and the duty is no less in a merged hospital:

> YES, I THINK the merger has helped us achieve our objectives. We've been able to do things we were unable to do before. We brought in better docs. We provide better care and have better checks and balances. We have been getting better marks from our employees. We get better marks from our marketing procedures. Our cash flow—everything—is more positive than it was before.
>
> [board chair, successful merger]

> I THINK THE positive thing from the merger is that we get to use the resources of both facilities. Each one has its strengths. For

instance, our partner hospital has a vice president of quality who brought both hospitals the benefit of that expertise. Likewise, our CFO is a computer genius, and our partner got the benefit of that.

[trustee, successful merger]

Executives realize the possible improvements that can result when once-separate organizations join. Additional personnel and services can be made available in ways that would not have been possible before the merger:

THE PARTNERSHIP WITH Hospital X has allowed us to bring new capabilities into the city, for example, senior citizen low-income housing. We'll have an expanded obstetrics presence, and the sponsors are now involved in a much larger organization with a much broader continuum of care than our hospital by itself ever had. Our hospitals are glued together; whether we can keep this afloat, I guess, is the key.   [CEO, financially struggling merger]

WHEN I FIRST came here, patient quality was not a focus. Our quality service was not a focus. Quality service is now a significant focus, and I think the level of caring has improved since the time of the merger.   [executive, successful merger]

Community representatives, likewise, have a stake in having the best healthcare services possible in their communities:

I THINK THAT the most positive aspect of the merger is that if it's able to work out properly, it should be able to provide better service and more affordable service.

[community representative, eventual failed merger]

I THINK THAT since the merger in the professional community there has been more credibility, understanding, and positive reaction.   [community representative, successful merger]

Persons inside the organization are no less interested in the prospects for future growth of their hospital. The additional opportunities for quality patient care that a merger presents are seen as reason to support the merger initiative:

FROM A CAREGIVER'S perspective, I think that we're better covering the county with consistent and quality services. For example, on weekends, the specialty surgeons can now cover each other from the two cities. And patients who need acute care can be sent to one hospital or the other. I think we have more services available now.
[employee, successful merger]

ONE BENEFIT OF the merger is the pooling of resources to try to provide better overall patient care. I think we now have maximum use of nursing staff and capabilities within the system.
[physician, financially struggling merger]

THE MOST POSITIVE thing about the merger would be the ability to provide optimum care for our patients and their families in the neighboring area. I would have to say that.
[employee, eventual failed merger]

The board chair in one of the more difficult, although successful, merger settings was a true leader and visionary. His merger had been in place for only two years, and he was able to recall the premerger days and one of the reasons why he got involved in all of the difficult and tedious meetings leading up to the merger itself:

IF YOU'D ASKED me our care philosophy five years ago, I'd have said it was quality care. But today it's higher-quality care.
[board chair, successful merger]

Hospitals exist for quality. No one connected with a hospital should sleep at night unless he or she feels certain that the care given in that hospital is supported by an infrastructure wholly focused on quality. Each of the mergers strove for that, even though not all were operationally successful.

A NEW WAY OF DOING THINGS

An organization's potential for new ideas is a function of its daily workplace atmosphere. Ideas and creativity are more likely to emerge in a climate of openness and trust than in an organization that is closed and stifling. A merged entity sits on the cusp of opportunity. Allowing creative approaches to flourish can make maximum use of the "doubled" people resources automatically available because of the merger. The merger voices share how this potential can be reached.

An ideal work force does not need bosses: all workers understand the business, understand their roles, and understand that they should do whatever it takes to further their business on a daily basis. Two comments indicate postmerger hospitals moving in this direction:

> WE'RE TRYING TO move in the direction of empowering people and enabling them, and we're building systems that will support that. We don't want people to check their brains at the door.
>
> [executive, successful merger]

> LET'S MAKE IT right for the customer—that's our outlook. So now we have more nurses actually taking the concerns and dealing with them up front rather than waiting for things to escalate to the point where the manager has to get involved.
>
> [employee, successful merger]

One of the mergers was able to adopt an entirely new way of dealing with labor unions. The board chair and CEO comment about this initiative, which reaped big dividends:

THE HUMAN RESOURCES executive sits down with bargaining units, tells it like it is, gives them goals, provides them with input, and lets them provide input. That process makes a tremendous difference for employees.   [board chair, successful merger]

WE'VE TAKEN A whole different approach to labor unions. We've gone to the unions and said, "You know, we're not here to bust any unions. We want you to be strategic business partners with us. We've got to make some changes, and you've got to help us come on board to make those changes." This is a cultural change. We've gone from really adversarial labor relations to an attitude of being strategic business partners.   [CEO, successful merger]

Although the following merger failed to stay together, its human resources executive had ambitious plans to reorganize her department to achieve rapid acceptance of their new partnership:

FROM A HUMAN resources perspective, as far as my department is concerned, one of the things I've told both staffs is that I'm going to co-mingle the cultures. We're going to take half the staff from here and half the staff from there, and we're going to mix them up. I hope to create little teams by function. If a benefits team, a labor relations team, and an employment team are co-mingled, they'll learn to work together with their team members in a whole different approach.   [executive, eventual failed merger]

Another merger needed to define its mission, and an all-inclusive process was carried out to accomplish that goal:

ONE OF THE first things we did was to put together our mission statement, create our core values. We did this with input from our board members, our volunteers, and our employees—probably 600 people or so had input to this mission statement.
          [executive, financially struggling merger]

A housekeeping worker was very excited about the entirely new approach taken when her supervisor was being hired:

> WE INTERVIEWED OUR new boss! That was kind of nice. Our director said, "I don't really know what kind of questions to ask him other than the business part, you know. You people can get more across to him than I probably could." So that has changed. It's changed a lot. [employee, successful merger]

Although what is new is not necessarily better, it is always different and often exciting. Organizations that do not want to embrace anything new will likely not venture into merger waters; those that do can be reenergized by the unlimited possibilities when new ideas are allowed to be introduced, tested, and evaluated. The difference between old and new is time; after new things are in place for a while, they soon become the new standard.

A BLEND OF THE BEST OF BOTH MERGER PARTNERS

To be able to look past the we-versus-they attitude and come together as true partners in a merger, hospital leaders and staffs must focus on doing what is best for their communities. Seeing excellence in a partner hospital's programs, services, and staff requires a hard look at the big picture, but the resulting synergy is powerful indeed. The merger voices capture the euphoria, as well as the difficulties, of achieving a blend of what is best about each merger partner.

Reciprocity is an important consideration, because a key strength of the merging organizations is their ability to complement each other:

> I THINK THE other hospital has things it can give us, just as we have things that we can give them. And I think that once we get past this newness it'll be really good.
>
> [employee, successful merger]

WE'RE TRYING TO capture the best of both worlds and create a blended culture. And cultural change is a very slow, slow process—painfully slow. [employee, successful merger]

WE'RE TOLD THAT with the merger, our hospital will still be able to exist. The partners have a lot of things to share with each other. It's a change, and we need to get the best of both our hospitals. I think we'll be able to provide better care as a team, joining the services. [employee, financially struggling merger]

THE SERVICES THAT the two hospitals offered were complementary. For example, we did not have nursing homes. Our partner hospital did. We had an extensive primary care and specialty physician practice network, and they really did not. We had some things in common, such as caring for the vulnerable population—we to the poor, and our partner hospital to the elderly and mentally ill. [executive, financially struggling merger]

Another realistic view is that the merged hospital organization needs to find the best practices available—whether from one or both of the merging hospitals or from outside the organization:

THE BIGGEST CHALLENGE, I would have to say, is bringing some symmetry to the organizations and doing the *right* thing. It's a challenge to not just say, "The Hospital X way is the right way, or the Hospital Y way is the right way"—actually doing an analysis and determining the principles behind things. We need to ask, "What should we be doing on this policy or this practice?" [executive, successful merger]

WE'VE WORKED VERY hard at blending cultures. Hospital X is the larger organization, Hospital Y is the smaller organization. There was always the tendency to say, "OK, we're going to do it like the larger hospital does, because that's the best way." We could see the people cringing when they heard that. Now we look at things and ask, "What is the best practice?" It may not be either hospital's practice, but we go out there and try to refine our databases.

[executive, successful merger]

The ability to appreciate the good things that each hospital brings to a merger is essential to its success. If the by-product of that analysis is eliminating duplications, the merger can come closer to its inherent operational efficiency goals:

WE'VE TRIED VERY hard to keep the unique qualities of each organization intact.   [executive, successful merger]

MERGING HOSPITALS CAN'T really compete—they have to join together. It's silly to have duplication of some services. In our department, for example, combining with the partner hospital's department was kind of nice; we got different ideas. We saw how the other department did things. That part was nice, too.

[employee, eventual failed merger]

Only when doctors are supportive of a hospital merger can success occur. Merging hospitals in the same community often have physicians who are members of both staffs. Physicians are huge stakeholders in the future of any hospital, merged or otherwise, and the ability to garner their support going forward takes respected leadership:

I GUESS THE biggest success is the participation of the doctors. It has sort of snowballed. Our ability to keep all the doctors at a very high level of participation has been a success.

[board chair, successful merger]

A doctor orignially from Eastern Europe offered perhaps the best insight about blending the best of both merger partners:

I COME FROM Hungary, and this merger is almost like the reunification of the two Germanys. There are a number of geographic and cultural differences, and it may take a long time before it will truly emerge as a single entity with a fairly uniform approach, philosophy, efficiency, and way of doing things.

[physician, successful merger]

A VIABLE PLAYER IN THE MARKET—THE MISSION ENDURES

A hospital with a long and proud history does not view entering a merger as putting a closed sign on the front door. They see a merger as one means to add to their security. Communities expect the mission of their local hospitals to continue after a merger, as do physicians and the staff who serve those hospitals. A merger that fulfills this expectation allows survival of the mission, as well as of the institution. The merger voices echo this hope for survival and an enduring presence.

One criterion indicating that an organization will probably survive is size. Two comments indicate that size was a factor in the success of their hospital mergers:

I THINK THE merger made us feel more secure because now we're not like a little sitting duck in a big pond, sitting there alone while things go on around us. We're all working for one thing. It gives me a sense of security that the hospital organization is making the right decisions for me, so I will have a job ten years from now.

[employee, successful merger]

THE ALLIANCE IS getting so big that it's tough to keep up with it. It's like having an organization with ten employees that all of a sudden has 50 employees. We don't know everybody as well as we knew the first ten.   [board chair, successful merger]

Keeping healthcare local is the prize for those mergers that came together with autonomy as one of their goals. Several persons appreciate what the continuation of local healthcare is doing for their communities through the mergers:

THE BOTTOM LINE is that we wanted to keep healthcare local, at the highest level, locally controlled and governed. And that was achieved instantaneously.　　　　　　　　　[CEO, successful merger]

I THINK THE consolidation itself is the biggest success. And again, we've earned the right—we put the organization in play. We didn't sell our organization to someone else. These are community resources, and they're not ours to sell or give up.

[CEO, successful merger]

THERE'S NOW A better cross-county referral. Because patients come into our merger organization, it helps keep a lot of business in the county and helps ensure our survival.

[physician, successful merger]

Preserving both mission and religious heritage was important to this community representative:

I AM FIRMLY convinced that without the coming together of the two hospitals, there would be no healthcare presence in the city today for our denomination. So that aspect of the merger is incredibly positive from my point of view. Everybody in the denomination leadership would say, "Thank God this has happened."

[community representative, financially struggling merger]

Two CEO's mirrored each other's sentiments about keeping their hospitals as viable players in the respective markets. Each pointed to the accomplishment of getting from premerger to postmerger according to their original plan:

WHAT WE SAID we would do—other than financial—after planning for it only a few months, we've done almost to every detail. We've had incredible support from the medical staff and on down the line. The whole thing is based on very difficult premises that the other systems in town haven't even begun to be willing to tackle. What we publicly said we would do, we did.

[CEO, financially struggling merger]

WE'VE BEEN ABLE to accomplish most, if not all, of the strategic initiatives we put together, plus ones that have come out of nowhere that we've had to deal with (some managed care issues, strategies, and so on).   [CEO, successful merger]

The hospital mergers in the communities of these interviewees have been very good and can be considered winners in many respects:

WE PUT THE merger together, and it's really working. It's really generating benefits. It's nice to stand back, smile, and say, "It is good, it can work, it is better than it was before." That's the good part.   [executive, successful merger]

YOU KNOW, THINGS were very competitive before the merger. So a lot of people going into it weren't sure how it was all going to work out. I think everyone's pleasantly surprised.

[executive, successful merger]

WHAT GIVES ME the most satisfaction about this alliance is that we've had a better financial picture at this hospital since we've had the alliance.   [employee, eventual failed merger]

I THINK THAT the merger organization has a great opportunity to achieve its goals, and it already is. I think that the target it's shooting for, which is a balance of clinical competence, local healthcare, and tertiary care, is a moving target, and its key role is to determine where that target is and then set systems up to make sure that it's followed.   [community representative, successful merger]

Finally, the most enthusiastic person commenting about surviving in the market so that the hospital's mission could endure was a CFO who had just had incredible offers by two third-party payers—all because of the synergy of the merger:

> I'LL ASK YOU pointedly, When was the last time you had an insurance company come into your organization and offer you an increase? The past two days we've had two insurance companies come to us and say, "Because of the network you built, and because of your location, we want to increase what we're paying you." This is the day, as CFO, that I've longed for. This is why we undertook this merger.   [executive, successful merger]

That is what everyone in hospitals everywhere longs for.

COMMUNITY-FOCUSED CARE

People involved in mergers are unanimous in saying that the communities are the true beneficiaries of the hard work involved in merging hospitals. Benefitting the community is the guiding principle and the ultimate prize. It is the yardstick by which hospital missions are judged and deemed worthy to continue.

Hospitals have an obligation to serve their communities well. Several comments note that very accomplishment, including a comment by an employee in a merger that continues to struggle, although not for any lack of purpose or effort:

> OUR GREATEST SUCCESS is the true recognition that both organizations have carried out their purpose—that of being quality care for their communities. Now we can successfully open a medical

clinic and not need to worry where that lab work will go or where the radiology will go, because we know it's going to be within the family somewhere. And we know that if there's a financial gain from that lab test, it can be reinvested back into our community.

[executive, successful merger]

I LIKE THE WAY it doesn't feel like competition anymore. At least in our community, it feels like we're working to do the right thing and working to really serve our customers well. We're not worrying about what Hospital X is doing or about what we are doing. We're worried about what the merger organization is doing as a whole! So I think that's a positive.   [executive, successful merger]

BOTH HOSPITALS ARE going to stay open, and people will still be able to receive their healthcare within one system. It may not be on this campus or that campus, but it will be within our system. So in the coming together our quality of service will just be better.

[employee, financially struggling merger]

The following trustees take their governance role very seriously when judging their hospitals' mergers and measuring themselves against the standard of representing the community interest:

ABSOLUTELY, IN MY opinion, the merger has achieved the objective of bringing together two long-time competitors so that the community's limited resources are not used for competition. Instead, they're used for delivering healthcare. The merger has preserved our mission to the poor; there's no question about that. Where we have not fulfilled the whole mission, I guess, is that the most efficient way to deliver clinical services has not been attained yet.   [board chair, eventual failed merger]

EVERYTHING IS LOOKED at from the perspective of the whole community. Not just whether the merger will do one hospital some good, or the other hospital, but the community, and the county as a whole.   [trustee, successful merger]

Another important aspect of community-focused care is access to services and convenience for patients. These comments underscore that commitment to those goals:

THE MERGER MAY make a lot of the older patients, especially, much more comfortable in knowing that their family member only has to come a few minutes as opposed to having to drive into the city and all of that.   [executive, successful merger]

I THINK THE merger is going to be better for everybody. I think it's great for the patients. It's easier in some ways for the patients to come out here to the central billing office. If they have a question about a bill, they can pull in here, they can park, and they can come in and talk to us. At the hospital it was very hard to find a place to park. This is more patient convenient. And we now have a shuttle bus that comes out here.
                              [employee, financially struggling merger]

WE CAN GIVE patients the service that they need, and they don't have to go further out. They can stay right here. And I feel we keep on growing. I really do. And that's what we want—for this place to stay open, keep our people, and make everybody happy.
                                    [employee, successful merger]

Because hospitals hold out the beacon of hope in a community, they must expect their merger decisions to be subject to close scrutiny. One community representative probed this line of thinking:

I THINK THE most positive thing to come out of the merger, far and away, is stewardship. The merger organization is not all the way there yet, you know, and it's a difficult position. They're between a rock and a hard place. Do we need two OB units? Do we need two surgeries? Do we need all this? And that is the kind of stewardship that has to happen. I mean, with the present state of healthcare and the tightness of reimbursement, stewardship is the key.

[community representative, successful merger]

One physician was quietly optimistic about his merger's ability to meet the needs of the community. Although he was supportive of the merger's purpose, he had seen other communities struggle unnecessarily with service consolidation:

I THINK THE best thing in a merger is a consolidation of services so there is less redundancy in providing things to the community.

[physician, successful merger]

The following inspiring comment comes from a community representative who was fully aware of the operational struggles in the hospital merger in his town but who felt an overpowering hopefulness that the turmoil was only temporary:

IN COMBINATION OF the two organizations, once it shakes out, I think we're going to have an organization that has values; cares about trying to give good service; and has a real continuation of the dedication to the poor, the helpless, and the homeless. That is needed. The new organization is going to articulate those goals, and they're going to try to achieve them. And to me, that's gold. That's really worth fighting for.

[community representative, financially struggling merger]

ASSESSING COMMUNITY PERCEPTION

Community reaction to, and perception of, a hospital merger varies. Perceptions may range from no reaction to a combat reaction.

The magnitude of the concept of merger begs for a magnitude of community views. The voices here relate perceptions in three categories: community support, community indifference or neutrality, and community antagonism.

Community Support

Positive and supportive community perceptions of a merger are shaped by a merger organization that works with the media to achieve press coverage that frames the merger in an accurately positive light. It is crucial that the new organization be explained to many constituencies, including the business community, and that the ethic of continued service to the community be shown through collaborative efforts by the two hospitals. These lessons come through clearly in the following voices:

> I THINK THE biggest success we have had is that everything we have done to date has received very, very positive press coverage. We could have been raked through the coals because of the perception that we were abandoning the community, but we've done a good job telling people what it is we're going to do and then actually doing it.   [executive, financially struggling merger]

> I WOULD SAY that I did not hear any negative comments from the public. It was all positive. I didn't hear anything negative from the medical staff at either hospital. It was all positive.
>   [executive, successful merger]

> PUBLIC REACTION TO the merger has been all positive. Two CEOs did a really nice job contacting people, such as the mayor, the county manager, the clergy, local councilmen—people who would really have an interest in it. People generally understand that Hospital X was in great jeopardy and that this merger was an attempt to preserve the services and the jobs in the area.
>   [executive, financially struggling merger]

WE HAVE A long list of accomplishments, including the overall community acceptance of the merger and the support we've received from the business community. We've had 100 percent of the business community's support for our doing this.

[CEO, successful merger]

I CAN'T HONESTLY say that any one person stood out as trying to bombard this merger or make it fail. I think there was more skepticism than anything else. No one specifically said that the merger wouldn't be any good or wouldn't work. No one said, "You guys don't know what you're doing." I never felt that.

[trustee, successful merger]

IT'S ALWAYS GOOD when two units work together. I think it's good for the area and good for the people, because it shows cooperation. It shows they can work together and probably save money. But that's not the important thing. The important thing is the service to the community.   [patient, eventual failed merger]

Community Indifference or Neutrality

Any merger entity can expect some indifference or neutrality in the community. How can something as sweeping in its effect on a community as a hospital merger be met with so little a reaction? The answer lies in human nature. People get interested in matters that directly affect them. Issues that appear too complex or too involved are largely ignored by the public, as these comments reveal:

OUR MERGER WAS met with deafening silence from the general public. Not word one. I still have yet, years later, to have someone come up to me and say, "That was a great thing you did," or "That was a stupid thing you did." The merger is just transparent to the general public. I don't think it matters to them.

[board chair, successful merger]

I DON'T KNOW that anybody really saw anything any differently. The other jointures in the metropolitan area certainly have been in the news enough, so the idea of hospitals joining does not surprise people.   [community representative, successful merger]

I SENSE PEOPLE saying, "Yeah, the healthcare world is changing. We don't understand it, but it's clear that people have to come together." Prior to this merger discussion, several hospitals had come together in a variety of different ways. So the community at large is saying, "Well, that's the way of the healthcare world at this moment in time."

[community representative, financially struggling merger]

I THINK THE community doesn't want to be abandoned and is probably unsure about two things: the quality of healthcare and the intent of the system. So I think you could characterize the community's thinking as a question mark: "Let's keep an eye on it and see how it plays out."

[community representative, financially struggling merger]

CERTAINLY WE ARE not (a) overly concerned or (b) even overly aware that the merger took place. And the only two places we've been are those two hospitals.   [patient, successful merger]

I CAN'T SEE that the merger makes too much of a difference for us. The only problem I have is our insurance. Hospital X accepts our coverage, but I don't think Hospital Y does, or maybe only on a referral-type basis. I mean, if hospitals are going to work together, the insurance they accept should coincide, too. That would help.

[patient, successful merger]

THE MERGER COULD be a very positive thing. I really don't know enough about it to give you a good answer.

[patient, eventual failed merger]

Community Antagonism

Along with positive and neutral reactions to a merger, of course, come feelings of antagonism from the community:

> WE'VE COME TO the conclusion that there is so much vested interest in the community that they don't really want any change that will affect them—job loss, physician income, those kinds of things. So I think that no matter what we did, we would get this negative reaction. The people in the community are not open to hearing what it is we're trying to achieve here. And that certainly does include the public officials, the mayor, many of the councilmen, and so forth.   [board chair, eventual failed merger]

> THE INNER CITY has lost its hospital now that the med/surg unit has moved and some other services will be moving next year. Many community residents see this as a local loss and not as something better in the suburbs.   [physician, financially struggling merger]

> I THINK THAT the people are just not listening. I think the merger is just too emotional a thing. Some politicians are quite vocal, saying, "We really need to save this hospital; it should be full-service." But the money's not there. There really are no other plausible solutions.
>   [community representative, eventual failed merger]

> THE BUSINESS COMMUNITY, as I would describe it—the professionals in the community—understood and accepted the consolidation plan. It was the middle of the pack—the nonprofessional people who haven't had the experience of running their own businesses and having to deal with the economics of business—who didn't understand and really didn't want to hear about merger. Once people began to disbelieve the numbers, it caught like a cancer. People gained comfort in saying, "The numbers aren't true,

so we don't listen to the numbers anymore." And they went right back to saying, "We don't like what you're doing to our hospitals."

[CEO, eventual failed merger]

I THINK THE mood in the community has been mixed. The community around this hospital campus—it is in the inner city and the poor neighborhood—is very frightened and very upset in thinking that they are losing their hospital. For example, the larger community is fearful that the emergency room is closing. That's not true, but the hospital organization needs to constantly get out there and say that.

[community representative, financially struggling merger]

WE WERE SERVING two distinct populations: an urban one and a suburban one. That very fact brought a great disruption and community outcry to us as we began to suggest moving clinical services in either direction.   [board chair, eventual failed merger]

IN ANY MERGER, I hate to see a loss of what is special about each place.   [patient, eventual failed merger]

Antagonistic comments from the community came only with struggling and failed mergers. These voices shared several lessons. First, people with vested interests do not budge from their positions easily, especially when they can garner support. Next, given the choice of staying with what we know or making a change, most of us will stay in familiar territory unless convinced that we have to change. Also, it is easier to focus on what would be lost due to a change rather than on something better that could be created. Finally, once again the interviewees demonstrated that perception is reality for most people, and perception is extremely difficult to change.

Both successful and less-than-successful mergers have an accurate understanding of what the mergers meant, provided, and represented in their communities: better healthcare, new ways of doing things, optimal blending of both merger partners, and ability to carry on the mission. The only dissimilarity between successful and less-than-successful mergers was that the successful mergers did not generate antagonism toward the merger organization.

What We Have Heard

Perception	Successful Merger	Less-Than-Successful Merger
A mecca of care and quality	yes	yes
A new way of doing things	yes	yes
A blend of the best of both merger partners	yes	yes
A viable player in the market	yes	yes
From the community		
Support	yes	yes
Indifference or neutrality	yes	yes
Antagonism	no	yes

Clues and Hallmarks

How much strength does community antagonism have in determining whether a merger will be successful? What does it really take to change perceptions? Given something as broad-based as a hospital merger, can neutral or negative perceptions even be changed? Or does the merger organization just have to move along and convince the skeptics over time that it is worthy of support?

Chapter 10

EVALUATING THE OUTCOME

IDENTIFYING WHAT SHOULD HAVE BEEN DONE DIFFERENTLY

The premise of case study learning is to examine an actual situation as an outsider in order to experience the circumstances "safely" and take away applicable lessons that apply to one's own situation and perspective. The beauty of studying what others do is that lessons can be learned that prevent not only "reinventing the wheel" but also duplicating costly mistakes. In studying a merger it is useful to both identity what should have been done differently and note the organization's secrets of success.

Communication

The study of mergers can teach much about successful communication. The merger voices share a lot about what they would have done differently to communicate about their mergers, because they all had to learn the hard way.

One communication failing was the inability to get the merger message out and across to people. There may have been a problem with the senders (lack of clarity, lack of explanation, or lack of effort) or a problem with the receivers (no one really cared, people heard but were not really listening, or the listeners were close-minded). This board chair and CEO were very frustrated when they talked with me:

WE NEVER WERE able to communicate to people that the acute care business is the business that's dying; the outpatient business is the business that's growing.

[board chair, eventual failed merger]

WE HAD A severe financial crisis, and we—all of us, including me—thought that the reality of the financial situation would carry the day. We thought that they—the community, the physicians, the employees—would look at the financial situation and say, "Sure, just do anything you need to do, because the financials are so bad." That didn't happen. Finances alone are not enough to sell a merger deal in a community and with the employers.

[CEO, eventual failed merger]

Getting the support of the medical staff was critical, and these hospital leaders felt that their efforts failed in that regard:

I BASICALLY THINK that the problem was a lack of education in the very initial stages, a lack of getting the medical staff involved and educating them on what an affiliation is. What is a merger, if that should occur? And what are the gives and takes? And what do we have to do, and how do we have to focus? And what kind of goals and objectives are we setting to look at that system? That education and communication was not in place.

[trustee, eventual failed merger]

ALTHOUGH THE MERGER ended up coming together pretty smoothly, I would have involved the medical staff more. Seeing it now, we should have anticipated the fringe groups within the staff and dealt with them more. As it was, we dealt mostly with those in the middle. There could have been less rancor if we had paid more attention to the entire spectrum of staff members and their ideas or concerns.   [physician, financially struggling merger]

I THINK I would have gotten medical executive committees together for the same type of education, dialog, and discussion. I
would have gotten the boards together to break the ice there and
really allow them to let their hair down and talk things out.

[trustee, eventual failed merger]

One board member experienced the onslaught of negative community attitudes toward his merger. He described how he would
have taken a much more proactive and challenging approach had
he been in charge:

I WOULD HAVE had community forums—many more community
forums. I would have talked to the dissidents; I would have gone
much more public. I have always had a very good relationship with
the press. I would never have said, "No comment." I would always
have said something. And I would have brought the press into the
merger the whole time.   [trustee, eventual failed merger]

A board chair pointed to the importance of early involvement
of community leaders to share the merger concept and garner
support. Even so, there was still room for improvement:

ONE OF THE first things the CEOs did together was speak to the
leaders of the communities. They met with the mayor, the executive
council, and the local assemblymen. I do feel they might have
missed the average citizens, though. But they also had the pastors
in and thought they were reaching many of the citizens through all
the church people, but that didn't work.

[board chair, financially struggling merger]

Two nurses in two very different merger situations mirrored
each other's comments regarding the degree of preparation their
staffs had during the mergers:

I THINK, PERSONALLY, I would have communicated more to my staff. I was well educated on the merger, I thought I got the information to the staff, but I don't know if I met all their goals and needs.   [employee, successful merger]

I WOULD HAVE gotten the nurses from the other hospital over here a lot sooner to start orienting them way back when we knew what was going to happen. I would have started the meetings, started getting them over here, and gotten them comfortable with our system before they came over and worked in it. It was pretty chaotic for a while, and I'm afraid patients suffered. I don't know any particular incidents, but there was a lot of confusion. It can be dangerous when you don't know where the crash cart is on the first day. It's scary. But things are settling now. They're learning; it's working; we'll be fine. It will work. But I think it could have been better, personally.   [employee, financially struggling merger]

The biggest problem in one merger that failed was the absence of a long-term plan. Due to the financial situation, the organization needed to make decisions quickly and neglected to see the larger picture or to communicate what it was doing. It would be interesting to note if leaders elsewhere could have done any better, given the circumstances:

TWO REALLY BIG failings of the implementation were that we sped it up too fast, and we didn't communicate ahead of time. In my opinion, we communicated our mission very poorly ahead of time. We didn't communicate why we were doing the merger and what the long-term benefit would be.

[board chair, eventual failed merger]

I WOULD HAVE not done the clinical consolidation as quickly. I would say that first we needed to communicate. We needed to have a plan in place to communicate what were doing, how we were doing it, so that when we announced that this clinical consolidation was coming, people would know what it meant. We needed to have a really good public relations campaign before that happened, and it was just not there.   [board chair, eventual failed merger]

The CEO in a successful merger offers a final comment about communication:

WE CAN NEVER communicate enough. We never get enough involvement in these processes. We can always do a better job of that.   [CEO, successful merger]

Culture

One of the overarching lessons that emerged from each of the mergers studied was that the merger organization did not consider corporate culture enough at the outset. Culture is manifested in two basic ways: (1) intrinsically, based in the fundamental beliefs and philosophies that underpin an organization and that have endured for years to give the organization its particular hallmarks (for example, "We are a family"), and (2) extrinsically, based in the ostensible practices, policies, and procedures that flow from the organization's deep philosophies (for example, "Because we are a family, employees get six days off for funeral leave for an immediate relative").

The merger voices relate their own struggles in coping with meshing cultures when hospitals merge. Two executives, each from mergers of opposite success poles, had similar feelings regarding the need to spend more time on, and pay more attention to, culture as a variable in the merged organizations they were creating:

IF I WERE to undertake a merger again, I would do a lot of the things the very same way. But I do not think we focused as much as we should have on establishing a new corporate culture. We should have created a new culture for this new entity, because really, the two hospitals are not what they used to be.

[executive, financially struggling merger]

I DON'T THINK we spent enough time in cultural variations within the organizations. Because there are fewer employees at Hospital X, they're a culture group. The folks at Hospital Y, even though they're nice, may not have some of the same closeness issues. I'd like to see more cultural evaluation about how we are going to bring people along, because I think those are some of the issues we're addressing today.   [executive, successful merger]

Time is more of a luxury than a commodity, both in personal life and in the daily life of a hospital merger, as this executive comments:

I THINK WE tried very hard to say, "We're going to create a whole new culture; we're going to try and take the best of the two merged hospitals." We found that was not going to work. What ended up happening was that just by the sheer fact that we had to get on with the everyday business of doing business, we had to take one culture and change it a bit. But we had to go in that direction. I think we were a little naive to say that we were going to create a whole new culture, because we just didn't have time to do that.

[executive, financially struggling merger]

This executive similarly reflects on the pragmatic approach to cultural considerations in a merger, which overtook the theoretical approach out of necessity:

I DON'T THINK we totally understood each other's culture before started. Once we came together and we started seeing the differences, that's when we tried to establish a new culture. It's a new organization. It's no longer Hospital X and Hospital Y; it's the merger entity, and that includes doctors' offices as well as the two hospitals. We developed a brand new team, a little different vision.

[executive, successful merger]

Merging organizations that can make the time to consider cultures as being two separate entities will be much more in tune with who they are and who they have been as organizations. They will also be much better prepared to create compatibilities among the work force members and various constituents.

Timing, Readiness, and Due Diligence

In the ideal world, there is plenty of time for everything. Nothing has to be rushed, so matters can be handled with the leisure that marks pondered, pensive decisions. Hospitals operate in anything but an ideal world, however. Time is usually of the essence: patient call lights should have been answered 20 minutes ago, a surgeon arrives early and demands to begin the procedure right away, a complex analytical report needs to be sent out to the board in the monthly mailing today, and employees expect feedback from managers the next day. That list can go on and on. And when things have to be hurried, readiness is usually lacking. The world of hospital merger decisions is not the ideal world, either, as our merger voices share.

The best time to move forward with a merger depends on the community. Local experts can be invaluable in helping a hospital evaluate if, and when, a hospital merger should proceed. These comments contain advice that is worth considering:

I WOULD SUGGEST that any board in any community really evaluate whether they're ready for this kind of relationship before they casually step into it. My guess is that most communities really aren't as ready as they think they are.

[CEO, eventual failed merger]

PERHAPS IF WE had a second chance to undertake the merger now, we would not necessarily need to be in as great a hurry as we were at that time. There is a classic example in another merger system: an organization that grows too fast can easily go into bankruptcy.   [physician, successful merger]

MANY PEOPLE HAVE told us we came in too soon as sponsors to be the savior and put the dollars on the table. If the employees had missed—for just one day—one payroll, we would have had immediate support and done it more correctly.

[trustee, eventual failed merger]

Whereas advice about timing and readiness for a merger must be community specific, advice about due diligence need not. Before a merger, painstaking and thorough due diligence is needed to make sure that all the decision makers fully understand the organizations that will be coming together. The following executives learned the hard way about the importance of due diligence and would undoubtedly pay more attention to it if time could be turned back:

I KNOW THAT from the start, we should have spent a lot more time, energy, and money doing a due diligence, because we just trusted people a little too much. After we got into this merger, the financial aspects and some of the issues on the financials weren't clearly stated, nor were they known until we got into the affiliation. We should have spent more time and not have been as trusting as we were. We ended up saying, "This deal has got to happen for the community. Let's make it happen." But we did not recognize that there could be some issues.

[executive, financially struggling merger]

ALL OF US may have been naive when we looked at the existing operations at this hospital. There were a significant number of write-offs related to things that were stuck on the balance sheet that people had hoped would happen but didn't happen. And I don't think we had a good handle on the margin on a lot of our outpatient business here.   [executive, financially struggling merger]

Governance

Governance is critically important to a hospital. Good governance is an expectation, whereas great governance is a luxury. In a merged hospital entity, routine hospital governance must rise to new levels to handle the scope of the decisions to be made and the prospects of shepherding an entirely new organization.

The merger voices share some important comments regarding their approaches to governance of merged entities. They also note areas for improvement. One executive pointed out that the boards of the merging hospitals should have gotten better acquainted before the merger:

I THINK I would have liked to have the boards meet together, probably over a three-month period, and act as if they were a system before they actually consolidated. Then they could have really gotten to know each other and how each other thought.
[executive, successful merger]

Several leaders, from successful and unsuccessful mergers alike, lamented the fact that at the outset of the mergers, the governance structure did not deal with board changes but tackled other consolidation issues instead. Not having unified boards in the beginning was seen as a real detriment and impediment to progress:

I THINK WE should have started out with a unified board from the very beginning. Then we would not have the mirrored board we have now. Our feeling was that, if we could not pull the governance piece together, we were not going to be able to stand in the community with any solidarity. That tore us apart in a way that I've never quite seen before.   [board chair, eventual failed merger]

I DON'T THINK the boards have really come together. There is a committee looking at board governance. A lot of things were done that needed to be done just to put the consolidation together. I think that's been disappointing.

[executive, successful merger]

WHAT ELSE COULD have been done? If you want to know where the difficulties are, where the troubles are, they're at the board level. Everything else is doing fine except the board. The board has a lot of trouble swallowing the merger because there are actually two separate boards, and each of them want to be in control. Now those boards are trying to integrate and become one smaller board.

[physician, successful merger]

FOR THE LAST year we have been in the midst of restructuring our governance to try to get one board from two. Truthfully, we have an unwieldy organization (Hospital X's board plus the system board), because that's how we've had to do it to get the deal done. We sort of shoehorned it all in together to make it happen, and we figured we'd fix it later. Now we're trying to fix it.

[board chair, successful merger]

IF I COULD do anything differently, I would have taken more time with the board structuring when we put it together so we wouldn't have to deal with it now. Maybe I'm just saying that because I'm dealing with it now! I don't think we did it right. We just did it in the expedient way, because if we hadn't done it that way, we probably wouldn't have gotten the deal done at all. But looking back, if we could have done it right then—sized the board correctly and had one board—I wouldn't have had the last two years of problems.

[board chair, successful merger]

Not having unified boards at the outset of the merger created a role conflict among the board members for this CEO:

> WE HAD THREE boards at the time, and they were beginning to determine what their whole role in the merger was. Were they advocates of the hospital? Or were they advocates of the system? Their default position was that they were advocates of their hospitals, because they were hospital boards.
>
> [CEO, eventual failed merger]

Finally, no board wants to be an impediment to progress and the attainment of merger goals. This CEO, however, noted that his postmerger board was concerned that it was not keeping up with the speed at which management needed to move:

> MAKE SURE THE board is nimble and in sync with management. In our situation, quite frankly, once management got its act together and began moving faster, it was almost as if the board became a drag on management. And that is the board's concern— that it is with management and able to support it and respond.
>
> [CEO, successful merger]

Premerger Work

The voices from mergers that would be considered less than successful agree that there is no substitute for concerted exploration of every single detail about a hospitals' operations before a merger is effected. The real skill lies in being able to visualize the newly merged entity at some point in the future and to anticipate its operational aspects. What premerger work needs to be done to accomplish that goal?

The interviewees overwhelmingly agreed that their premerger work should have focused on the quality of the due diligence process. They also should have scrutinized the financial assumptions rather than merely accepting (or not questioning) them. There was great frustration and disappointment in the voices of each of these persons in regard to premerger financial work, and they chided themselves for not questioning their assumptions about the financial situation more thoroughly:

THERE WERE THINGS that were not handled properly. For instance, three different due diligences by three different groups of attorneys asking for three different sets of information three different ways was not the most ideal way to handle things from all the different departments. The stress level was tremendous. It was not planned very well. It created more stress.

[executive, eventual failed merger]

THE FINANCIAL FEASIBILITY study and the due diligence should have been done in a traditional, exacting way, as opposed to operating off of assumptions and things like that. I think a lot of good faith went into the merger early on, a lot of accepting things on face value. Given that, there have been an awful lot of surprises.

[executive, financially struggling merger]

I THINK THE problems that we're having financially have to do with the quality of the work we got from the consultant. Also, mergers—like combat—never work the way they were planned. Adjustments are always needed. I wish we had had a better plan for one of the hospital buildings, to make it useful faster. That would have helped us financially. When hospital-based consultants are hired, they don't think in terms of that. They just think about hospital services and moving them around.

[executive, financially struggling merger]

I WOULD HAVE examined the feasibility study and the depth of financial issues here much more if I had been the sponsors and the consultant. They're unburying things now, and it's too late. The shovel's in the ground; the money's lost. So I would go back and be more careful about the depth of that analysis.

[board chair, financially struggling merger]

WHAT I'M DISAPPOINTED in, and the board is disappointed in, is the original assumptions. Yes, it was the consultants who did the feasibility study, but they based it on information management gave them. So who had the wrong assumptions? Was management too optimistic? Were they not realistic? So I can't blame the consultants, because they based their studies on the information given to them, and they didn't get good information.

[board chair, financially struggling merger]

WHEN WE DID the due diligence, we spent almost a million dollars, so the problem was not a lack of due diligence. But we had a set of financial statements that had been signed off by auditors. Well, we were not going to go back and test their assumptions. However, when we got to the closing, the consultant, auditors, and even the sponsors came back and said, "Wait a minute, we think some of the assumptions on revenues might be flawed."

[CEO, financially struggling merger]

Related to the quality of due diligence is the quality of pre-merger planning for the overall campuses, which after a merger will consist of two locations/facilities instead of just one. Several interviews mentioned master facility planning as a key issue they would address better if they could do things over again:

WE DIDN'T ANALYZE thoroughly enough what was going to happen on this campus and how were we going to stay prominent in the community.   [employee, financially struggling merger]

I THINK THE role of this particular campus would need to have been looked at again.   [physician, financially struggling merger]

WE REALLY DON'T have a good plan for what this hospital building is going to be when it grows up. Instead of trying to look at the
building as it is, an acute care facility, we finally realized, "Why
don't we call it what it is?" It's going to be an inner-city healthcare
service delivery location. I think defining it that way is going to be
very useful. So I have hopes that we're going to turn this facility into
something that's going to have some survivability potential.

[community representative, financially struggling merger]

THE SYSTEM COULD become viable if we could get that drain of a
hospital building off our backs financially and convert it into at
least something that handles its own overhead. I think that we're
going to have to do some more sandpapering of our souls before
we know what that is.   [executive, financially struggling merger]

Although speed is not always the greatest virtue, to this executive
speed made the difference between a continued financial struggle
to operate and a more positive financial position that would provide a comfortable cash stream as the rest of the merger unfolded:

I THINK IF we could do it differently, we'd probably do a lot of
things faster. I think we would probably have spent more time
doing what we haven't done—trying to figure out what this facility
and this community want and need. I think we might have moved
the med/surg beds sooner. And we might have handled the physician practice and the hospital-based physicians differently.

[executive, financially struggling merger]

Overall, premerger planning about service lines and locations
was seen as desirable—and lacking—by one nurse, who was dis-
gusted with what she perceived as the leaders' "constant mind
changing" on essential decisions that affected her life—and of
everyone else's:

BEFORE ANYONE ANNOUNCED any type of merger, everything should have been settled. There were a lot of unanswered questions. There were no concrete plans that the administrator or anyone else could tell the employees or the community. It seemed like there was so much opposition. The organization changed plans along the way, and that was even more confusing to the public.

[employee, eventual failed merger]

Two employees from mergers that had less-than-positive outcomes would have begged the leaders to request more input and participation from those who would be affected by the decision to merge. One of these speakers, a nurse, was offended that decisions were being made by board members who "only set foot in the place once a month for meetings," whereas employees who spent hours there, day after day, were given no voice or role in one of the most important decisions to affect her hospital:

IF I WERE in charge, I would have obtained more input from the employees as far as how they felt their department ran, how they thought we could merge, and any suggestions. I think that before I'd make any drastic move such as a merger, I would want to talk to the people who would be directly handling these things and ask how they felt about the merger before making the move.

[employee, eventual failed merger]

THE ADMINISTRATION COULD have taken a bit longer. They should have realized that the decision they made affects people. They were not going to be affected by the decision; the people were. And I don't think they have a clue about that. You know, you need to involve the people—certainly the department heads. The lower management echelon are really the ones catching the brunt of the decisions, because they're in the middle. They're getting it from on high, and they're getting it from down under. And they're in the middle. Those are the people who I think should have been involved a great deal more.   [employee, financially struggling merger]

Leadership

Good executive leadership is essential in any hospital. In creating a merged hospital organization, one of the initial decisions is selecting the CEO. Are there incumbents at both hospitals? Are both worthy of consideration? If not, how can the CEO selection create the best outcome? The merger voices address what they would have done differently in regard to executive leadership.

Two executives expressed as their main frustration the fact that needed adjustments were not made to the leadership team at the outset. Executives from the two merging hospitals stayed on—some in different, expanded, or created roles—and this hampered progress toward the merger goals:

> I THINK I would have immediatley tackled some of the senior management issues. It was a painful year. While we did OK, we didn't do as well in the first year as we could have. We made up a lot of ground in the second year.   [executive, successful merger]

> FROM THE HUMAN resources side, we didn't do enough to create a homogeneous leadership team. And we're paying for it now.
> [executive, financially struggling merger]

One physician who vigilantly watched the merger developments from his administrative post lamented the myriad problems that surfaced in the merger because of inadequate leadership by the executive staff. He was sad as he talked about this missed opportunity, which he felt was lost for good:

> AS A COMBINED administrative team, we were not strong enough to say to the board, right from the beginning, "You know what? This is why you hired us. We're the experts in healthcare. And we're

going to give you our best plan." What we did was sort of take a side seat and let the three different boards go at it. We didn't take much of an active role in trying to straighten them out. Eventually, the board felt they were now the experts in what was best for the community, best for the medical staff, and best for the two institutions. They sort of took things into their own hands, and what the administration was saying took a second seat.

[physician, eventual failed merger]

A similar sentiment was expressed by an equally sad executive who, in hindsight, would have taken a much more active role himself in getting the concept of leadership in front of his peers:

I DON'T BELIEVE we did as good a job as we should have in leadership development, or learning how to fully exercise communication and support amidst the management of the whole organization—not just one side or the other. Based on early efforts to make the leadership absolutely lead as well as be an active player in day-to-day decision making, I'd say we could have had a significant impact on success.   [executive, financially struggling merger]

NOTING SECRETS TO SUCCESS

Vision

There is something to be said for selecting a pathway, for whatever reasons, and then not straying no matter what. Every merger starts with well-intentioned goals and expectations. One of the secrets to success is remaining faithful to those goals.

One board chair never wavered from his determination to stay focused on the community served:

I THINK THAT as we move forward, we have to constantly remember where we came from—and where we want to go. We don't want to sell out the community.   [board chair, successful merger]

The financial struggles of their merger gave two executives much pause for thought and reanalysis of plans. However, they remained firmly committed to the plans developed and never veered from the original vision:

> I THINK OUR strength is our ability to implement the strategy by reconfiguring the services using both substantial hospital plants. We have a great system. In other places, some of these things blow up: the physicians or the staff are going bonkers, the CEOs don't work together, things are called off, or the boards hate each other. Not here.   [executive, financially struggling merger]

> OTHER THAN MISSING our financial targets, we're doing what we said we wanted to do, because it was the right thing to do. It's just happening. We haven't veered from plan.
>   [CEO, financially struggling merger]

A successful merger involves strategic planning. In the following cases, the original vision laid the groundwork for success to follow once the merger was fully operationalized:

> WE WANTED TO undertake this merger early on while we were still strong and not compete with one another. We didn't waste dollars. And our strategy was not to circle the wagons to keep competition out. It was to circle the wagons so we could compete. A merger takes a tremendous amount of vision and understanding. It wasn't easy to do.   [CEO, successful merger]

> WE ARE NOW in a strong position in relation to any insurance company. We can say, "We represent all the doctors, so many beds, and a larger service area. If you want to negotiate, you can sit down and talk to us." That's where the system, the merger, really bears fruit.   [CEO, successful merger]

Communication of goals is essential in any merger, but one physician was especially complimentary about the communication provided to medical staff members. He was unwavering in his commitment to the success of the merger because of that communication:

THE REASONS FOR the merger were very clear to the physicians, the financial situations of both facilities were very clear to the physicians, and the commitment of the hospitals to provide quality care on an ongoing basis was very clear. I think that facilitated the support by the physicians.

[physician, financially struggling merger]

Finally, a patient reminds us that carrying out its mission should be the top goal of any hospital:

ABOVE EVERYTHING ELSE, keep the care of your people on top, your utmost importance. And forget all the politics and everything else that enters into the picture.

[patient, eventual failed merger]

Leadership

Good leadership, by both the board and the administrative staff, is an essential catalyst to bring about the changes demanded in a hospital merger situation. Several executives and physicians attributed the ability of their merger to move forward and accomplish goals to one individual: their organization's CEO. Great times make great leaders, and these comments indicate the respect for the CEO in hospital mergers:

OUR MERGER'S SUCCESS was due to the early appointment of the CEO. That sort of cut out any question, or at least allowed him quickly to plan and give direction. It gave him the ability to put together an organization chart that really got us moving quickly.

[executive, financially struggling merger]

AT FIRST THERE was a wave of anxiety, because mergers always involve downsizing; people lose their jobs. Our CEO got past that. He made himself available. He had meetings for hours and hours on end to discuss everything. He assured us that the merger was to secure our future. It will make the system stronger; we will save money; we will have more money to expand other services. That's security. So he sold the employees on the merger very quickly. And now people are willing to go across campus to have jobs.

[physician, successful merger]

THE CEO WAS the fuse. For two years the boards met together, physicians met together, department heads talked. The merger almost fell apart; people said it was never going to happen. And then there was an agreement to pursue it.

[physician, successful merger]

WE HAD A CEO, one person who said, "This is what we're going to do. We have a vision, and here's where we're going to go." We had a plan, and we had people, particularly the CEO, who made us all accountable to hitting some of those things.

[executive, financially struggling merger]

One CEO who was not able to keep his merger together offers another thought about leadership at the board level:

DON'T EVER TRY to run these systems with multiple levels of governance. Don't ever try it. We knew it a year ago, and we learned the same lesson that all the other health systems have learned over and over: it is essential to have one governance structure; having multiple governance levels just doesn't work.

[CEO, eventual failed merger]

It is clear from the viewpoints expressed regarding an evaluation of the merger outcome that successful mergers show marked differences compared to less-than-successful mergers. Governance, leadership, communication, and due diligence stand out as key aspects contributing to those differences. While focusing on goals is common to all the mergers, including those that are less than successful, it is clear that several other factors must align to create success.

What We Have Heard

Factor	Successful Merger	Less-Than-Successful Merger
Communication	yes	no
Culture fit	yes	no
Timing, readiness, and due diligence	yes	no
Governance effectiveness	yes	no
Premerger work	yes	no
Leadership	yes	no
Vision	yes	yes

Clues and Hallmarks

Some hospital mergers are influenced by urgency of acting—money is running out. How can this be managed so that a *best* outcome is achieved and just not the most expedient?

Physician and employee buy-in is essential, yet at some point information needs to be handled in a strategic or even confidential manner. When do you tell whom? Is it possible to start over with culture in a merged organization, eliminating all traces of the partners' respective cultures?

Chapter 11

REPLAYING THE TAPE

The wisdom from these merged hospitals has sounded. The voices have been many and the viewpoints eclectic. It is useful to summarize those viewpoints that were expressed by voices from the successful mergers compared to those from the less-than-successful mergers. The following table gives that comparison and can serve as a reference outline for the advice and experiences shared in this book.

Putting All the Lessons Together

	Successful Merger	Less-Than-Successful Merger
Why Organizations Merge		
Avoid takeover and survive	yes	yes
Retain autonomy	yes	yes
Create efficiencies and provide better care	yes	yes
Stop competing	yes	yes

(continued on following page)

Putting All the Lessons Together
(continued)

	Successful Merger	Less-Than-Successful Merger
What Organizations Expect to Accomplish		
Improve quality and expand services	yes	yes
Provide for the community and maintain autonomy	yes	yes
Eliminate competition and work together	yes	yes
Survive, continue in the mission, decrease costs, gain market share	yes	yes
How Hospitals Fit Together		
Discovering greater alignment than expected	yes	yes
Discovering greater differences than expected	yes	yes
Building trust, considering culture, and overcoming past grievances	yes	yes
Comparing partners financially premerger	yes	yes
Achieving financial strength from the merger	yes	no
Experiencing financial weakness from the merger	no	yes
Governance Structure		
Superboard	yes	no
Single board	no	yes
Mirror boards	no	yes
Consolidated board in discord	yes	no
Postmerger Conditions		
Communication		
• Open	yes	no
• Adequate	yes	no
• More than before merger	yes	no
• Frequent	yes	no
Medical staff link		
• Cross-credentialing	yes	yes
• Joint activities	yes	no
• Physicians supportive	yes	no
• Physician concern about clinical consolidation	no	yes

	Successful Merger	Less-Than-Successful Merger
Department consolidations	yes	yes
Infrastructure consolidations	yes	yes
Workload and teamwork	yes	yes
Positive perceptions of care	yes	yes
Fallout		
• Less of a family feeling, more impersonal	yes	yes
• Difficulty achieving acceptance	yes	yes
• Lack of planning	yes	yes
• Uncertainty and staff outmigration	yes	yes
How Merged Organizations Handle Employees		
Avoid staff reductions	yes	no
Increase job opportunities	yes	yes
Give more autonomy	yes	yes
How Merged Organizations Are Perceived		
A mecca of care and quality	yes	yes
A new way of doing things	yes	yes
A blend of the best of both merger partners	yes	yes
A viable player in the market	yes	yes
Perceptions from the community		
• Support	yes	yes
• Indifference or neutrality	yes	yes
• Antagonism	no	yes
How Merged Organizations Evaluate the Outcome		
Communication	yes	no
Culture fit	yes	no
Timing, readiness, and due diligence	yes	no
Governance effectiveness	yes	no
Premerger work	yes	no
Leadership	yes	no
Vision	yes	yes

To close, here are some final thoughts from our merger voices that offer additional words of advice:

GOALS

Remember the hospital's point of origin, be faithful to the community, and always focus on patient care.

"Circle the wagons" to compete, not to keep the competition out.

BOARD

Get the board solidified quickly.

Make sure the board is nimble and synchronized with management.

Get good information, make a decision, stick to that decision, and be strong enough to take the flack.

Mirror boards work; avoid thinking of the board as we versus they.

Keep the board in the same room; do not let factions meet on their own.

Have the board ask, "Are we ready to merge?"

MEDICAL STAFF

Remember that physician involvement makes all the difference.

At least 50 percent of the physicians must accept the merger for it to succeed. They must understand why the merger is being contemplated, what the financial situations are, and how the hospitals are committed to providing ongoing quality patient care.

LEADERSHIP

Appoint the CEO early to ensure consistent direction and coherent planning.

Realize that the CEO is the key to success.

Get a cohesive management staff as quickly as possible.

Take the surgical approach to management consolidation: consolidate early and swiftly.

OPERATIONS

Remember that geography causes competition, but geography is also a hospital's greatest strength.

Downsize when consolidations occur.

Call it a merger after "small" things, such as joint purchasing, have been implemented.

FINANCES

Be impeccable in exercising due diligence.

In a merger, time lines are twice as long, financial losses are twice as big, and too much optimism can be fatal.

COMMUNICATION

Talk it out.

Keep searching for ways to inform better and do everything better.

Share information completely, freely, and openly.

Forget the hospital name; use the merger name and the new identity.

Remember that inpatient care is dying and oupatient care is growing.

SUPPORT/TRUST

Keep in mind that some people will never support the merger, no matter what.

Realize that change—and merger acceptance—is a personal issue.

Be thorough, give it time, and go through the hoops.

Build bridges and relationships ahead of time.

Remember that a financial crisis alone is not enough to sell the deal among the members of the community and employers.

Suggested Readings

American Hospital Association. 1990. *Mergers, Acquisitions, and Consolidations: A Checklist for Success*. Chicago: American Hospital Association.

Arvey, R. D., T. J. Bouchard, Jr., N. L. Segal, and L. M. Abraham. 1989. "Job Satisfaction: Environmental and Genetic Components." *Journal of Applied Psychology* 74 (2): 187–92.

Bader, B. S. 1997. "Look Before You Leap." *Trustee* March, 18–22.

Barney, J. B. 1986. "Organizational Culture: Can It Be a Source of Sustained Competitive Advantage?" *Academy of Management Review* 11 (3): 656–65.

Barton, J., and S. Folkard. 1991. "The Response of Day and Night Nurses to Their Work Schedules." *Journal of Occupational Psychology* 64 (2): 207–18.

Bartunek, J. M., and M. K. Moch. 1987. "First-Order, Second-Order, and Third-Order Change and Organization Development Interventions: A Cognitive Approach." *Journal of Applied Behavioral Science* 23 (4): 483–500.

Bauman, R. P., with P. Jackson and J. T. Lawrence. 1997. *From Promise to Performance: A Journey of Transformation at SmithKline Beecham.* Boston: Harvard Business School Press.

Beach, L. R. 1997. *The Psychology of Decision Making: People in Organizations.* Thousand Oaks, CA: Sage.

Bellandi, D. 1998. "Deal Deluge." *Modern Healthcare* 28 (5): 24.

———. 2000. "Spinoffs, Big Deals Dominate in '99." *Modern Healthcare* 30 (2): 36–44.

Benedict, R. 1934. *Patterns of Culture.* Boston: Houghton Mifflin.

Brooks, G. R., and V. G. Jones. 1997. "Hospital Mergers and Market Overlap." *Health Services Research* 31 (6): 701–22.

Buono, A. F., with J. L. Bowditch and J. W. Lewis, III. 1985. "When Cultures Collide: The Anatomy of a Merger." *Human Relations* 38 (5): 477–500.

Campion, M. A. 1988. "Interdisciplinary Approaches to Job Design: A Constructive Replication with Extensions." *Journal of Applied Psychology* 73 (3): 467–81.

Cartwright, S., and C. L. Couper. 1993. "The Role of Culture Compatibility in Successful Organizational Marriage." *Academy of Management Executives* 7 (2): 57–70.

———. 1995. "Organizational Marriage: 'Hard' vs 'Soft' Issues." *Personnel Review* 24 (3): 32–42.

Chandran, J. P. 1994. "The Impact of Mergers and Acquisitions on Organizational Culture." Ph.D. diss., University of South Florida. Ann Arbor, MI: UMI Dissertation Services.

Chatterjee, S. 1998. "Are Related Mergers Really Better? A Research Note." Presented at the Academy of Management national meetings, July.

Chatterjee, S., with M. H. Lubatkin, D. M. Schweiger, and Y. Weber. 1992. "Cultural Differences and Shareholder Value in Related Mergers: Linking Equity and Human Capital." *Strategic Management Journal* 13 (2): 319–34.

Cooke, R. A., and D. M. Rousseau. 1988. "Behavioral Norms and Expectations: A Quantitative Approach to the Assessment of Organizational Culture." *Group and Organization Studies* 13 (3): 245–73.

"Corporate Culture: The Hard-to-Change Values That Spell Success or Failure." 1980. *Business Week* Oct. 27, 148–60.

Czarniawska, B. 1997. *Narrating the Organization: Dramas of Institutional Identity.* Chicago: University of Chicago Press.

Deal, T. E., and A. A. Kennedy. 1982. *Corporate Cultures: The Rites and Rituals of Corporate Life.* Reading, MA: Addison-Wesley.

Deloitte & Touche. 1997. *Hospital Market Update* 1 (Nov. 10).

Denison, D. 1996. "What is the Difference Between Organizational Culture and Organizational Climate? A Native's Point of View on a Decade of Paradigm Wars." *Academy of Management Review* 21 (3): 619–54.

Deshpande, R., J. V. Farley, and F. E. Webster, Jr. 1993. "Corporate Culture, Customer Orientation, and Innovativeness in Japanese Firms: A Quadrad Analysis." *Journal of Marketing* 57 (Jan.): 23–37.

Drennan, D. 1992. *Transforming Company Culture: Getting Your Company from Where You Are Now to Where You Want to Be.* London: McGraw-Hill.

Eberhardt, B. J., and A. B. Shani. 1984. "The Effects of Full-Time vs Part-Time Employment Status on Attitudes Toward Specific Organizational Characteristics and Overall Job Satisfaction." *Academy of Management Journal* 27 (4): 893–900.

Flannery, T. P., and J. B. Williams. 1990. "Management Culture and Processes." *Healthcare Forum Journal* 33 (4): 52–57.

Fox, M. L., D. J. Dwyer, and D. C. Ganster. 1993. "Effects of Stressful Job Demands and Control on Physiological and Attitudinal Outcomes in a Hospital Setting." *Academy of Management Journal* 36 (2): 289–318.

Frost, P. J., L. F. Moore, M. R. Louis, C. C. Lundberg, and J. Martin (eds.). 1991. *Reframing Organizational Culture.* Newbury Park, CA: Sage.

Furnham, A. 1992. *Personality at Work.* London: Routledge.

Geertz, C. 1973. *The Interpretation of Cultures.* New York: Basic.

Giddens, A. 1994. *Central Problems in Social Theory: Action, Structure and Contradiction in Social Analysis.* Berkeley, CA: University of California Press.

Hale, D. G., and R. L. Johnson. 1998. "Deals That Could Not Close—Or Shouldn't Have." Paper presented at the NHLA/AAHA Conference, Jan. 15–16.

Herzberg, F. 1968. "One More Time: How Do You Motivate Employees?" *Harvard Business Review* 46 (Jan./Feb.): 53–62.

Hofstede, G. 1980. *Cultures Consequence's: International Differences in Work-Related Values.* Beverly Hills, CA: Sage.

Hofstede, G., and B. Neuijen, D. D. Ohayu, and G. Sanders. 1990. "Measuring Organizational Cultures: A Qualitative and Quantitative Study Across 20 Cases." *Administrative Science Quarterly* 35 (2): 286–316.

Hunt, J. G., and A. Ropo. 1995. "Multi-Level Leaderships Grounded Theory and Mainstream Theory Applied to the Case of General Motors." *Leadership Quarterly* 6 (3): 379–412.

Hutchins, E. 1996. *Cognition in the Wild.* Cambridge, MA: MIT Press.

James, L. R., L. A. James, and D. K. Ashe. 1990. "The Meaning of Organizations: The Role of Cognition and Values." In *Organizational Climate and Culture,* edited by B. Schneider, 40–84. San Francisco: Jossey-Bass.

Jermier, J. J. 1991. "Critical Epistemology and the Study of Organizational Culture: Reflections on *Street Corner Society.*" In *Reframing Organizational Culture,* edited by P. J. Frost, L. F. Moore, M. R. Louis, C. C. Lundberg, and J. Martin, 223–33. Newbury Park, CA: Sage.

Kippley, J. F. 1994. *Marriage Is for Keeps.* Cincinnati, OH: The Foundation for the Family.

Kitching, J. 1967. "Why Do Mergers Miscarry?" *Harvard Business Review* 45 (Nov./Dec.): 84–101.

Kotter, J. P. 1978. *Organizational Dynamics and Intervention.* Reading, MA: Addison-Wesley.

Kotter, J. P., and J. L. Heskett. 1992. *Corporate Culture and Performance.* New York: Free Press.

Kunda, G. 1992. *Engineering Culture: Control and Commitment in a High-Tech Corporation.* Philadelphia, PA: Temple University Press.

Likert, R. 1967. *The Human Organization: Its Management and Value.* New York: McGraw-Hill.

Lincoln, Y. S., and E. G. Guba. 1985. *Naturalistic Inquiry.* Newbury Park, CA: Sage.

Lowery, J. E. (ed.). 1997. *Culture Shift: A Leader's Guide to Managing Change in Health Care.* Chicago: American Hospital Publishing.

Lutz, S. 1996. "Failed Mergers Offer Valuable Lessons." *Modern Healthcare* 26 (1): 54–55.

MacEachern, M. T. 1935. *Hospital Organization and Management.* Berwyn, IL: Physicians' Record.

Martin, J. 1992. *Cultures in Organizations: Three Perspectives.* New York: Oxford University Press.

"Merger Results a Letdown to Execs." 1996. *Trustee* Sept. 3, 3.

Mirvis, P. H., and A. L. Sales. 1990. "Feeling the Elephant: Culture Consequences of a Corporate Acquisition and Buy-Back." In *Organizational Climate and Culture*, edited by B. Schneider, 345–82. San Francisco: Jossey-Bass.

Morrison, E. W., and S. L. Robinson. 1997. "When Employees Feel Betrayed: A Model of How Psychological Contract Violation Develops." *Academy of Management Journal* 22 (1): 226–56.

Nahavandi, A., and A. R. Malekzadeh. 1988. "Acculturation in Mergers and Acquisitions." *Academy of Management Review* 13 (1): 79–90.

O'Malley, S. 1996. "Lessons from Mergers That Failed to Click." *Health System Leader* July, 4–13.

Park, S. H., and G. R. Ungson. 1997. "The Effect of National Culture, Organizational Complementarity, and Economic Motivation on Joint Venture Dissolution." *Academy of Management Journal* 40 (2): 279–307.

Pettigrew, A. M. 1979. "On Studying Organizational Culture." *Administrative Science Quarterly* 24 (4): 570–81.

Ramaswamy, K. 1997. "The Performance Impact of Strategic Similarity in Horizontal Mergers: Evidence from the U.S. Banking Industry." *Academy of Management Journal* 40 (3): 697–715.

Reichers, A. E., and B. Schneider. 1990. "Climate and Culture: An Evolution of Constructs." In *Organizational Climate and Culture*, edited by B. Schneider, 5–39. San Francisco: Jossey-Bass.

Robinson, M. 1996. "Health Care Becomes Big Business." *Business and Health* 14 (1): 29–32.

Rollins, T. 1993. "Two Studies Define Link Between Corporate Culture and Business Performance." *Employee Relations Today* 20 (2): 141–57.

Rodat, C. 1994. "Hospital Mergers and Affiliations." *Health System Leader* June, 4–13.

Rousseau, D. M. 1990. "Assessing Organizational Culture: The Case for Multiple Methods." In *Organizational Climate and Culture,* edited by B. Schneider, 153–92. San Francisco: Jossey-Bass.

Sackmann, S. A. 1991. *Cultural Knowledge in Organizations: Exploring the Collective Mind.* Newbury Park, CA: Sage.

Salipante, P. F. 1992. "Providing Continuity in Change: The Role of Tradition in Long-Term Adaptation." In *Managing the Paradoxes of Stability and Change,* edited by S. Srivastva and R. E. Fry, 132–67. San Francisco: Jossey-Bass.

Salipante, P. F., and K. Golden-Biddle. 1995. "Managing Traditionality and Strategic Change in Nonprofit Organizations." *Nonprofit Management and Leadership* 6 (1): 3–20.

Sandrick, K. M. 1996. "What 'Ya Know?" *Trustee* May, 26–29.

Saxton, T. 1997. "The Effects of Partner and Relationship Characteristics on Alliance Outcomes." *Academy of Management Journal* 40 (2): 443–61.

Schein, E. H. 1991a. "The Role of the Founder in the Creation of Organizational Culture." In *Reframing Organizational Culture,* edited by P. J. Frost, L. F. Moore, M. R. Lewis, C. C. Lundberg, and J. Martin, 14–25. Newbury Park, CA: Sage.

————. 1991b. "What Is Culture?" In *Reframing Organizational Culture,* edited by P. J. Frost, L. F. Moore, M. R. Louis, C. C. Lundberg, and J. Martin, 243–53. Newbury Park, CA: Sage.

————. 1992. *Organizational Culture and Leadership.* San Francisco: Jossey-Bass.

————. 1996. "Culture: The Missing Concept in Organization Studies." *Administrative Science Quarterly* 41 (2): 229–40.

Schmitt, N., B. W. Coyle, J. K. White, and J. Rauschenberger. 1978. "Background, Needs, Job Perceptions, and Job Satisfaction: A Causal Model." *Personnel Psychology* 31 (4): 889–901.

Schneider, B. (ed). 1990. *Organizational Climate and Culture.* San Francisco: Jossey-Bass.

Schneider, B., J. K. Wheeler, and J. F. Cox. 1992. "A Passion for Service: Using Content Analysis to Explicate Service Content Themes." *Journal of Applied Psychology* 77 (5): 705–16.

Schutz, W. C. 1958. *FIRO: A Three-Dimensional Theory of Interpersonal Behavior.* New York: Rinehart.

Selznick, P. 1957. *Leadership in Administration: A Sociological Interpretation.* New York: Harper & Row.

Sherer, J. L. 1994. "Corporate Cultures: Combining Disparate Corporate Cultures at Merged Hospitals." *Hospitals and Health Networks* 28 (9): 20–26.

Shirley, R. C. 1977. "The Human Side of Merger Planning." *Long Range Planning* 10 (1): 35–39.

Shortell, S. M., J. L. O'Brien, J. M. Carman, R. W. Foster, E. F. X. Hughes, H. Boerstler, and E. J. O'Connor. 1995. "Assessing the Impact of Continuous Quality Improvement/ Total Quality Management: Concept Versus Implementation." *Health Services Research* 30 (2): 377–401.

Singh, J., W. Verbeke, and G. K. Rhoads. 1996. "Do Organizational Practices Matter in Role Stress Processes? A Study of Direct and Moderating Effects for Marketing-Oriented Boundary Spanners." *Journal of Marketing* 60 (July): 69–86.

Smircich, L. 1983. "Concepts of Culture and Organizational Analysis." *Administrative Science Quarterly* 28 (3): 339–58.

Spector, P. E. 1997. *Job Satisfaction: Application Assessment, Cause and Consequences.* Thousand Oaks, CA: Sage.

Tichy, N. M. 1983. *Managing Strategic Change: Technical, Political and Cultural Dynamics.* New York: Wiley.

Trice, H. M. 1991. "Comments and Discussion." In *Reframing Organizational Culture*, edited by P. J. Frost, L. F. Moore, M. R. Louis, C. C. Lundberg, and J. Martin, 298–308. Newbury Park, CA: Sage.

Trice, H. M., and J. M. Beyer. 1993. *The Cultures of Work Organizations.* Englewood Cliffs, NJ: Prentice-Hall.

Tylor, E. B. 1924. *Primitive Culture: Researches into the Development of Mythology, Philosophy, Religion, Language, Art, and Custom.* New York: Brentano's.

Vestal, K. W., and S. W. Spreier. 1997. "Facilitating Change Through Cultural Assessment." In *Culture Shift: A Leader's Guide to Managing Change in Health Care,* edited by J. E. Lowery, 15–38. Chicago: American Hospital Publishing.

Weber, Y. 1996. "Corporate Cultural Fit and Performance in Mergers and Acquisitions." *Human Relations* 49 (9): 1181–202.

Weick, K. E. 1995. *Sensemaking in Organizations.* Thousand Oaks, CA: Sage.

Wernimont, P. F., P. Toren, and H. Kapell. 1970. "Comparison of Sources of Personal Satisfaction and of Work Motivation." *Journal of Applied Psychology* 54 (1): 95–102.

Wilkins, A. L. 1983. "The Culture Audit: A Tool for Understanding Organizations." *Organizational Dynamics* 12 (2): 24–38.

Wilkins, C. A. 1996. "An Ethnographic Study of the Emergence of Culture in Two Merging Health Organizations." Ph.D. diss., Ohio University. Ann Arbor, MI: UMI Dissertation Services.

Witalis, R. W., and J. McLeod. 1984. "The Process and Management of Corporate Consolidations." *Hospital Forum* 27 (2): 20–22.

Wolf, M. G. 1970. "Need Gratification Theory: A Theoretical Reformulation of Job Satisfaction/Dissatisfaction and Job Motivation." *Journal of Applied Psychology* 54 (1): 87–94.

About the Author

Sister Nancy Linenkugel, OSF, EDM, FACHE

Sister Nancy Linenkugel, OSF, EDM, FACHE, has been president and chief executive officer (CEO) of Providence Hospital since 1986 and president and CEO of the Providence Health System since its founding in 1987. Both organizations are located in Sandusky, Ohio. Prior to coming to Sandusky, Sister Nancy was vice president of support services at St. John Medical Center, Steubenville, Ohio, from 1980 to 1985, after completing a graduate degree in healthcare administration. She is a Fellow of the American College of Healthcare Executives (ACHE), and is serving as a member-at-large on its Board of Governors until 2004. Previously, she served as the elected ACHE Regent for Northwestern Ohio. Sister Nancy served as a junior high school teacher for seven years prior to entering healthcare.

Sister Nancy has a BA in education from Mary Manse College, Toledo; a master's degree in hospital and health administration from Xavier University, Cincinnati; and a doctorate in management from the Weatherhead School of Management, Case Western Reserve University, Cleveland.

She has served on numerous community and academic boards, including serving as president of the Erie County Chamber of Commerce, the Sandusky Rotary Club, and the Board of Leadership Enrichment and Development Sandusky (LEADS). She has also received significant professional and community service awards, including being inducted into the Ohio Women's Hall of Fame in 1999 and being named 1 of 12 "Up and Comers" nationally for 1990 by *Modern Healthcare* magazine. She was the 1990 national runner-up for the Young Healthcare Executive of the Year Award from the ACHE, and she was Erie County's Businesswoman of the Year in 1992, receiving the ATHENA Award.

She is a church organist and a cellist with various groups, including a national orchestra of healthcare personnel. Sister Nancy has been a member of the Sisters of St. Francis, Sylvania, Ohio, since 1968.